THE LIMBIC SYSTEM

ANATOMY, FUNCTIONS AND DISORDERS

NEUROSCIENCE RESEARCH PROGRESS

NEUROSCIENCE RESEARCH PROGRESS

THE LIMBIC SYSTEM

ANATOMY, FUNCTIONS AND DISORDERS

RUSSEL T. GEARY
EDITOR

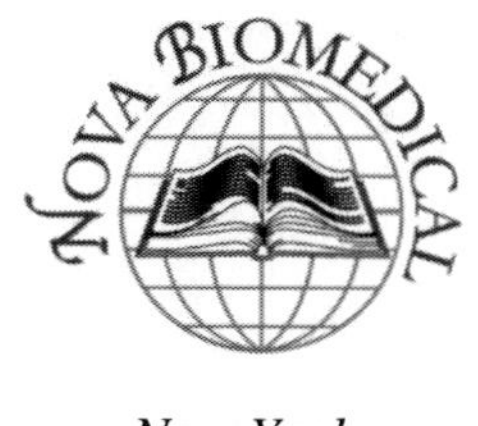

New York

Copyright © 2014 by Nova Science Publishers, Inc.

For permission to use material from this book please contact us:
Telephone 631-231-7269; Fax 631-231-8175
Web Site: http://www.novapublishers.com

NOTICE TO THE READER

The Publisher has taken reasonable care in the preparation of this book, but makes no expressed or implied warranty of any kind and assumes no responsibility for any errors or omissions. No liability is assumed for incidental or consequential damages in connection with or arising out of information contained in this book. The Publisher shall not be liable for any special, consequential, or exemplary damages resulting, in whole or in part, from the readers' use of, or reliance upon, this material. Any parts of this book based on government reports are so indicated and copyright is claimed for those parts to the extent applicable to compilations of such works.

Independent verification should be sought for any data, advice or recommendations contained in this book. In addition, no responsibility is assumed by the publisher for any injury and/or damage to persons or property arising from any methods, products, instructions, ideas or otherwise contained in this publication.

This publication is designed to provide accurate and authoritative information with regard to the subject matter covered herein. It is sold with the clear understanding that the Publisher is not engaged in rendering legal or any other professional services. If legal or any other expert assistance is required, the services of a competent person should be sought. FROM A DECLARATION OF PARTICIPANTS JOINTLY ADOPTED BY A COMMITTEE OF THE AMERICAN BAR ASSOCIATION AND A COMMITTEE OF PUBLISHERS.

Additional color graphics may be available in the e-book version of this book.

Library of Congress Cataloging-in-Publication Data

ISBN: 978-1-63117-993-8

Library of Congress Control Number: 2014939497

Published by Nova Science Publishers, Inc. † New York

Contents

Preface

The primary cortical areas that we include under the umbrella of limbic system include the olfactory cortex, amygdala and hippocampal formation, and nearly all parahippocampal cortex and cingulate cortex, but also caudal orbital and medial prefrontal cortex and part of the temporal polar cortex, and the ventral part of the agranular and dysgranular part of the insular cortex. It should be noted that researchers still disagree on how many and which areas exactly comprise the limbic system, however, most agree that it includes the hippocampus, subicular cortex, parahippocampal cortex, cingulate cortex, septal nuclei, basolateral amygdala, mammillary bodies, the anterior thalamic nuclei and their interconnections and connections. Subcortical areas, such as the cortical and central amygdala, the septal nuclei, and diencephalic regions, including the mammillary bodies and the anterior thalamic nuclei, make up the rest of the limbic system. The limbic system is highly interconnected, both by direct connections and by indirect projections through diencephalic regions such as the mammillary bodies and the anterior thalamic nuclei. This book discusses the areas of the limbic system which play a role in epilepsy; chronic musculoskeletal pain; the effects altered gravity may have on the limbic system; and finally, the affects opioid addiction has on the limbic system.

Chapter 1 – Many areas of the limbic system play a role in epileptogenesis, one of the main epileptogenic areas within the limbic system is the hippocampus. The hypothesized relation between hippocampal formation damage and epileptic seizures dates back to the early 19th century, and by 1880 Sommer had clearly identified an area of the hippocampus proper (i.e., Sommer's sector or area CA1) which was consistently damaged in the epileptic patients that he studied. Several subsequent reports have supported the idea that, in patients with temporal lobe epilepsy, the epileptogenic focus is in the hippocampus proper in the majority of patients, and that limited resection of the hippocampal focus can often abolish subsequent seizure activity.

However, other areas of the medial temporal lobe, especially the amygdala and entorhinal cortex, have also been shown to be the origin of epileptic foci in a significant number of cases.

Chapter 2 – Emotions are often cited as a potential cause of musculoskeletal symptoms. However, the explanations given for this relationship are frequently vague and non-specific. This chapter focuses on the specific mechanisms by which the limbic system can influence musculoskeletal symptoms. A conceptual framework is presented suggesting conscious and sub conscious interpretation of emotional responses to events can impact all systems of the body generating or modifying musculoskeletal symptoms. The limbic system can directly modify the activity of the autonomic, endocrine, immune and musculoskeletal systems. Through these systems it is able to alter the activity of all other systems. In addition the limbic system is integral to our psychology which can similarly modify symptoms. It is important to note that multiple systems are being affected simultaneously. The end result may be that pain is felt in a specific region, which can be viewed within the context of current knowledge on pain physiology and the neuromatrix. An understanding of these processes may improve a clinician and patient's understanding of what may be influencing symptoms. It is hoped this understanding may help improve outcomes.

Chapter 3 – Changes in gravity conditions have often been shown to affect vestibulo-cerebellar functioning. In the present review, the authors describe recent experiments indicating a role for hypogravity and hypergravity on limbic system functioning. The effects of spaceflight on the limbic system include changes in cell diameter and monoamine levels as well as immediate early gene products. A method to determine the effects of hypogravity while earthbound is the hindlimb unloading response in rodents. Like spaceflight, hindlimb unloading causes changes in neuropeptide levels and cell stress responses. To gauge the complete actions of gravity changes, hypergravity induced by acceleration of caged but freely moving rodents placed inside a centrifuge has been examined. Notable changes include altered mRNA levels of several genes expressed in the hippocampus. These results are discussed in the context of interactions between vestibulo-cerebellar areas and the limbic system under changes in gravity conditions.

Chapter 4 – Anterior cingulate cortex, amygdala and insular cortex are characterized by very high concentration of mu-opioid receptors, and enkephalin is the most abundant opioid agonist in these limbic system structures. Neuroimaging studies of healthy subjects consistently showed activation of limbic cortex and subcortical structures after mu-opioid agonist injection, and involvement of opioid innervation of limbic structures into generation of positive emotions, control of pain and negative emotions. Experimental and clinical studies demonstrated that chronic administration of pharmacological opioid agonists induced profound remodeling of brain structures supporting reward and emotion processing. Chronic opioid treatment strengthened interneuronal connections involved into opioid-seeking behaviors, whereas processing of non-drug-related rewards and emotions is deficient in addicted animals and humans.

In: The Limbic System
Editor: Russel T. Geary

ISBN: 978-1-63117-993-8
© 2014 Nova Science Publishers, Inc.

Chapter 1

The Limbic System Plays a Significant Role in Epilepsy

*Larry Ver Hoef[1], Inga Kadish[2]
and Thomas van Groen[2,3]*
[1]Department of Neurology, UAB Epilepsy Center,
University of Alabama at Birmingham,
Birmingham, AL, US
[2]Department of Cell, Developmental and Integrative Biology,
University of Alabama at Birmingham,
Birmingham, AL, US
[3]Department of Neurobiology,
University of Alabama at Birmingham,
Birmingham, AL, US

Abstract

Many areas of the limbic system play a role in epileptogenesis, one of the main epileptogenic areas within the limbic system is the hippocampus. The hypothesized relation between hippocampal formation damage and epileptic seizures dates back to the early 19th century, and by 1880 Sommer had clearly identified an area of the hippocampus proper (i.e., Sommer's sector or area CA1) which was consistently damaged in the epileptic patients that he studied. Several subsequent reports have supported the idea that, in patients with temporal lobe epilepsy, the epileptogenic focus is in the hippocampus proper in the majority of patients, and that limited resection of the hippocampal focus can often abolish subsequent seizure activity.

However, other areas of the medial temporal lobe, especially the amygdala and entorhinal cortex, have also been shown to be the origin of epileptic foci in a significant number of cases.

Introduction

It has been shown that many areas of the limbic system play a role in epilepsy, with one of the main areas involved in epileptogenesis being the hippocampus. The observed relation between hippocampal formation damage and epileptic seizures dates back to the early 19th century [1]. By 1880 Sommer had clearly identified an area of the hippocampus proper (i.e., Sommer's sector or area cornu Ammonis 1or CA1) which was consistently damaged in the epileptic patients that he studied (Sommer, 1880 [2]). The so-called "hippocampal sclerosis" typically demonstrates a pattern of preferential neuronal loss and astrogliosis both in the CA1 and CA4 (a.k.a end-folium area or hilus) subfields more than in the CA3 subfield and granule cell layer of the dentate gyrus, and little to no neuronal loss in the CA2 subfield. Recent reports have strongly supported the idea that, in patients with temporal lobe epilepsy (TLE), in the majority of patients the epileptogenic focus is in the hippocampus proper, and that therefore resection of the hippocampal focus will often abolish subsequent seizure activity. In many patients, analysis of the degree of hippocampal sclerosis compared to the frequency and severity of epileptic activity gives a strong indication that the damage to the hippocampus was present before the initial epileptic activity. It has been demonstrated that especially the pyramidal neurons in field CA3 of the hippocampus are contributors to the initiation of epileptic seizure activity and are damaged by recurring seizures.

However, it should be noted that while the hippocampus is the main area of epileptogenesis, other areas of the medial temporal lobe, especially the amygdala and entorhinal cortex, have also been shown to be the origin of epilepsy in a significant number of cases.

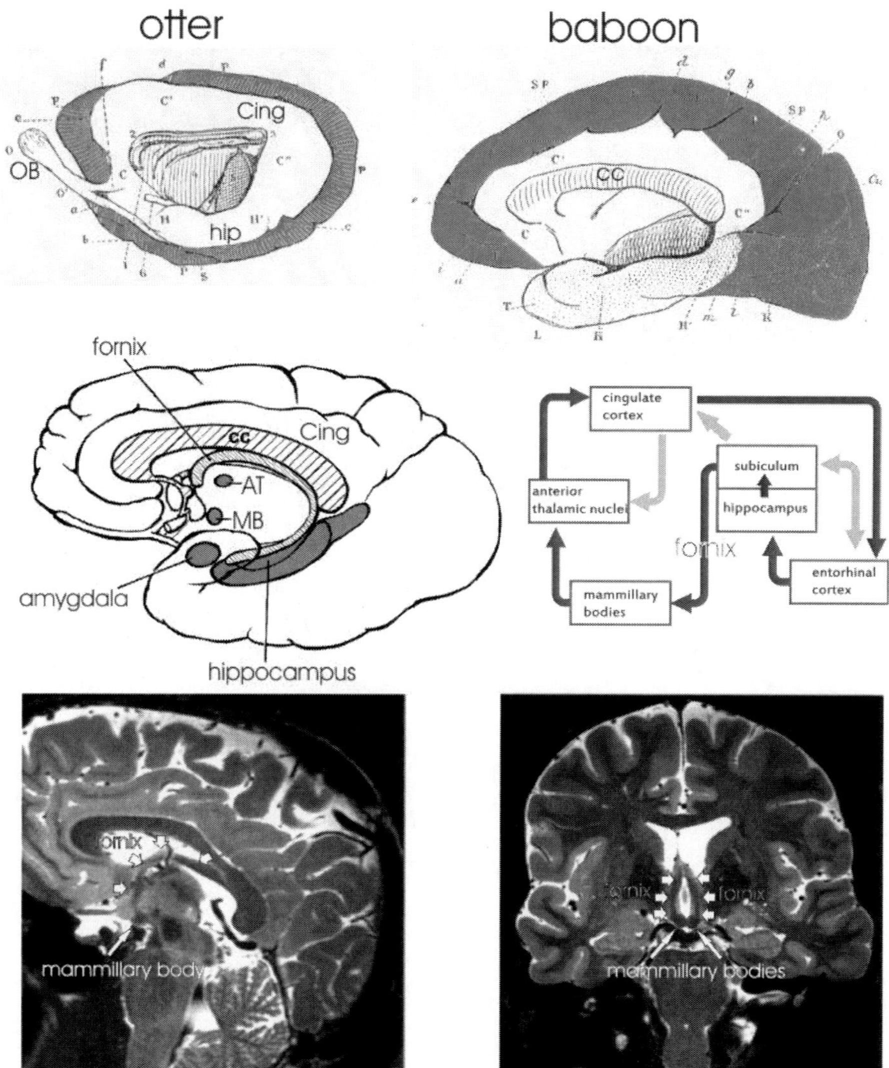

Figure 1. Three sets of two images showing the limbic lobe of Broca, the Papez ciruit and the MRI anatomy of the Papez circuit, respectively. Top, the limbic lobe of Broca is shown in the otter and the baboon, note the connection of the limbic lobe with the olfactory system in the otter. Center, the Papez circuit as it is present in the human brain, and a schematic representation of the "real" Papez circuit, the lighter arrows depict the reciprocal connections within the Papez circuit. Bottom, two MRI images of the fornix and mammillary bodies in the human brain. AT-anterior thalamic nuclei, cc-corpus callosum, Cing-cingulate cortex, hip-hippocampus, MB-mammillary bodies.

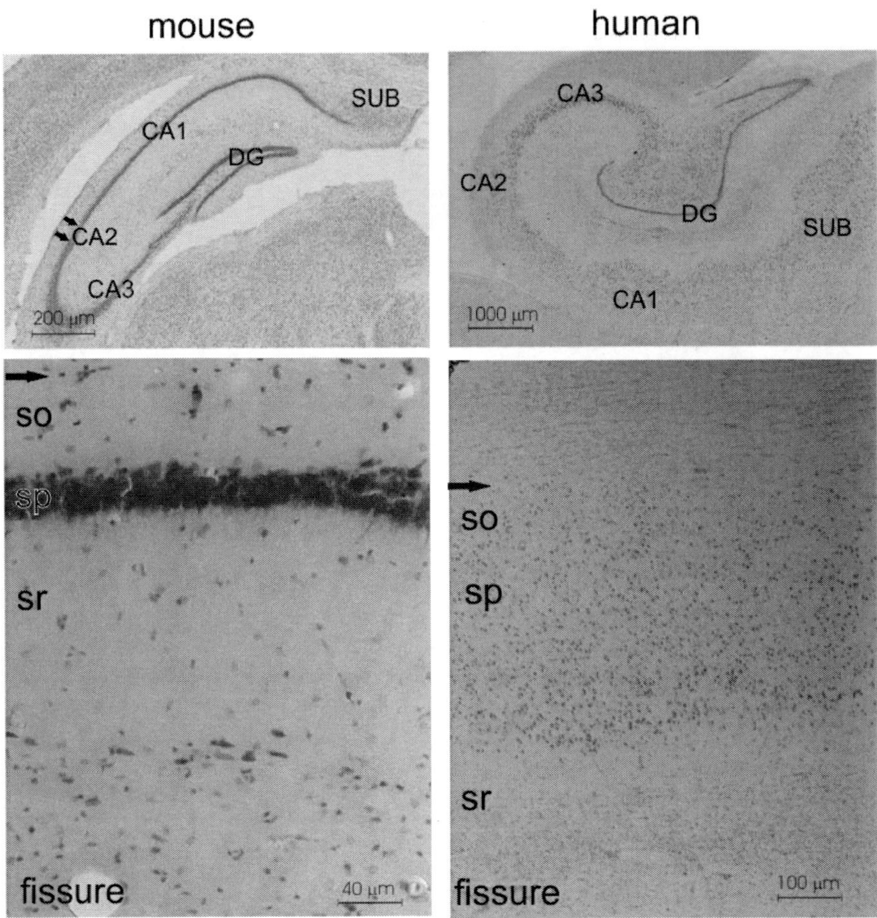

Figure 2. Two low power and two high power images of the mouse (left) and human (right) hippocampus. CA1-area cornu Ammonis 1 CA2-area cornu Ammonis 2, CA3-area cornu Ammonis 3, DG-dentate gyrus, so-stratum oriens, sp-stratum pyramidale, sr-stratum radiatum, SUB-subiculum. The arrow indicates the border between stratum oriens and the corpus callosum.

History of the Neuroanatomy of the Limbic System

The history of the anatomical term "limbic" for brain regions is quite long; the first person the use the term was Willis (1664 [3]) who named the cortical regions that form the medial edge of the telencephalon as limbus (i.e., border in Latin). Much later, Broca (1878 [4]) was the first to use the designation of this area of cortex as "Le grand lobe limbique", or "the great limbic lobe". Broca's great limbic lobe comprises the gray matter areas that lay as the transition between the neocortex and the diencephalon (i.e., the cingulate, hippocampal, olfactory, and parahippocampal cortices) and that together form a circle on the medial edge of the hemisphere (Figure 2). The limbic lobe is rostrally connected to the olfactory bulb (Figure 2, otter) and is smaller in microsmatic ("low" sense of smell) animals and bigger in macrosmatic ("high" sense of smell) animals. Together, these observations indicated to Broca that the main function of the limbic lobe was likely related to olfaction. Later, several researchers expanded on this view even to the point of suggesting that the limbic lobe was a pure "smell brain" or rhinencephalon [5]. By the 1940's, research suggested that these regions of limbic cortex also received other types of sensory information and were possibly involved in other functions, especially emotion [6].

In 1937 Papez [7] hypothesized that there was an anatomical basis for emotions. Based on the existing anatomical knowledge, and on earlier proposals on the anatomical basis of emotional functioning, he proposed an anatomical circuit that showed how emotional experiences would lead to the expression of emotions. The circuit is now known as the Papez circuit (Figure 2), which consists of a "circuit" of connections between limbic cortical areas and the diencephalon. Papez's [7] original hypothesis was that the cingulate cortices together with the hippocampal formation received a major input from sensory areas of the cerebral cortex and that the hippocampal formation processed this information and projected this to the mammillary bodies (part of the hypothalamus) from which the appropriate emotional response could be coordinated. The circuitry of these connections has been elucidated in more detail and it is now clear that the afferent and efferent connections of the hippocampal formation are far more varied and complex than Papez's original model (Figure 2). Two years after Papez hypothesis, Klüver and Bucy [8] demonstrated that extensive lesions to the temporal lobe that damaged significant parts of the limbic lobe (including the amygdala, entorhinal cortex and the hippocampal formation) profoundly influenced the affective behavior of subhuman primates. On the basis of Klüver and Bucy's and other studies, MacLean (1952 [9]) suggested that the term limbic system should be applied to the limbic lobe areas. MacLean emphasized that the limbic system elements (which now also included the amygdala) were at the interface between somatic and visceral areas of the brain. The limbic system could thus relate these two systems to each other and to the ongoing behavior of the animal. For that reason he envisioned the limbic system functioning as a "visceral brain". Nauta (1979 [10]) further expanded on the definition of the limbic system by showing that many areas of the limbic cortex were directly connected to the hypothalamus and brainstem. Thus, the limbic system is a concept that has undergone considerable redefinition since its original introduction as "limbus" [11]. Finally, although the individual limbic areas are functionally diverse, serving emotional responses on the one hand, and learning and memory on the other, the high degree of interconnectivity strongly suggests that these areas likely also do have an underlying unity.

Neuroanatomy of the Limbic System

The primary cortical areas that we include under the umbrella of limbic system include the olfactory cortex, amygdala and hippocampal formation (including the subicular cortices), and nearly all parahippocampal cortex and cingulate cortex, but also caudal orbital and medial prefrontal cortex and part of the temporal polar cortex, and the ventral part of the agranular and dysgranular part of the insular cortex. It should be noted that researchers (e.g., [11]) still disagree on how many and which areas exactly comprise the limbic system, however, most agree that it includes the: hippocampus, subicular cortex, parahippocampal cortex, cingulate cortex, septal nuclei, basolateral amygdala, mammillary bodies, the anterior thalamic nuclei and their interconnections and connections. Subcortical areas, such as the cortical and central amygdala, the septal nuclei, and diencephalic regions, including the mammillary bodies and the anterior thalamic nuclei, make up the rest of the limbic system. The limbic system is highly interconnected, both by direct connections and by indirect projections through diencephalic regions such as the mammillary bodies and the anterior thalamic nuclei (through the fornix and mamillothalamic tract; Figure 3). Despite the fact that the concept of the limbic system is based on historical and developmental principles, and that it consists primarily of relatively "simple" allocortex and transitional cortex, it is not a "primitive" part of the brain. Even though the limbic cortical and subcortical areas appear phylogenetically early (for instance, the hippocampus is designated as a part of the archicortex, i.e., "ancient cortex"), many limbic areas of cortex reach their greatest development in human. For example, compared to primary sensory and motor cortices, the entorhinal cortex expands more in size from lower mammals to humans (Figure 3; [12]). Accordingly, these areas should not be seen as antiquated remnants, but they are brain regions that have continued to develop both structurally and functionally throughout phylogeny. Limbic structures such as the hippocampus (and septum) are clearly more advanced in higher primates and man than in "low" species such as insectivora [12]. In contrast, olfactory structures (olfactory bulb and olfactory cortices) are clearly smaller in "higher species", such as primates, compared to insectivores (for instance, in the hedgehog the olfactory related cortical structures encompass more than 50% of the brain). These opposite trends imply the existence of two functional systems within the limbic system (the olfactory system and the memory/emotion system[s], [13]) being predominantly independent of one another [12]. Even if it is quite clear that these two systems do significantly interact, as is demonstrated by the famous "madeleine memory" of Proust.

Within the hippocampus the greatest phylogenetical changes are found in hippocampal area CA1, with the enlargement of area CA1 being the highest in humans. In phylogenetically "low species" such as hedgehogs the pyramidal layer of area CA1 is very dense and narrow, in mice it is already slightly wider and slightly less dense (Figure 1). In man (and most primates) the pyramidal neurons are dispersed over the whole of stratum oriens and reach the alveus (Figure 2). Similarly, the enlargement of the entorhinal cortex (EC) is accompanied by structural differentiations which are reflected both in laminar and regional complexity [14].

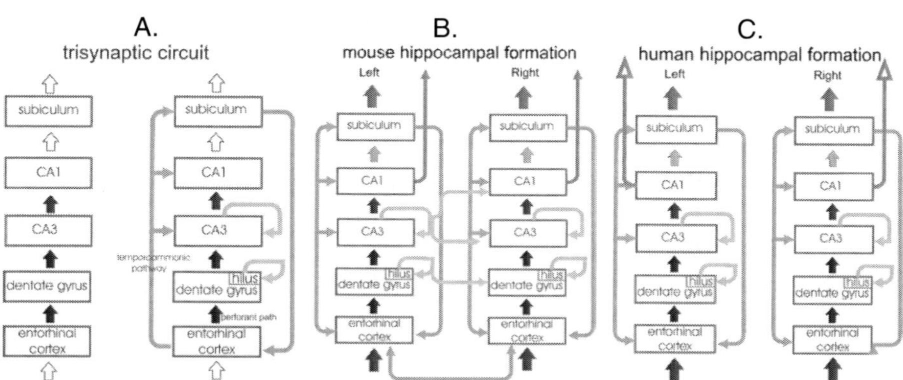

Figure 3. Three sets (A-C) of schematic diagrams of the trisynaptic circuit in the hippocampus. A, left, original concept of the trisynaptic circuit, right, anatomically correct concept of the trisynaptic circuit (in the mouse). B. the trisynaptic circuit of the mouse with the commissural connections within the hippocampus added. C. the trisynaptic circuit of the human with the commissural connections within the hippocampus added, note the lack of commissural connections. CA1-area cornu Ammonis 1,CA3-area cornu Ammonis 3.

In mice and rats, in general, only medial and lateral entorhinal cortex are distinguished, even if more modern studies recognize 5 regions (which are subdivisions of the lateral and medial entorhinal cortex; REF), in contrast in human entorhinal cortex has been subdivided into anything from eight [15] to 16. The subdivisions of the entorhinal cortex have different connections and receive distinct inputs [16], and are therefore assumed to subserve different functions. In most mammals only the lateral entorhinal cortex receives an olfactory input [17, 18], whereas the medial entorhinal cortex receives more processed infoprmatioon through the perirhinal and postrhinal cortices [16, 19].

On the basis of neuroanatomical studies, the entorhinal cortex is regarded as the relay station that provides the major source of afferent input to the hippocampus. –It should be noted that several subcortical inputs (e.g., septum, locus coeruleus, raphe nuclei) project to all areas of the hippocampus.- The perforant path input to the dentate gyrus arising from layer II neurons in the entorhinal cortex has traditionally been regarded as the major pathway by which information is transferred (Figure 3A). The lateral and medial perforant path (originating in layer II cells of the lateral and medial entorhinal cortex, respectively) form synapses on the outer and medial molecular layer of the DG, which in turn corresponds to the distal (outer) and the intermediate parts of the dendrites of dentate granule cells. It should be noted that the inner part of the molecular layer of the dentate gyrus receives both intrinsic connections from the hilar neurons, and extrinsic input from the supramammilary nucleus. The perforant path input to the dentate gyrus arising from layer II neurons in the entorhinal cortex has traditionally been regarded as the major pathway by which information is transferred to the hippocampus (Figure 3). However, more recent studies have demonstrated that other elements of the perforant path that project directly to CA3 and CA1 (i.e., the temporoammonic pathway) are more important than thought previously (Figure 3), and that the properties of different neuronal elements in the entorhinal cortex may determine the way in which information is passed on to and processed by the hippocampus. Furthermore, anatomical and functional data also indicate that the parahippocampal region, which is comprised of the perirhinal (PC), postrhinal (POR) and entorhinal cortices, is an essential link between neocortex and hippocampus [19]. For instance, lesion studies have demonstrated that memory functions previously ascribed to the hippocampus actually depend on the integrity of the rhinal cortices [20].

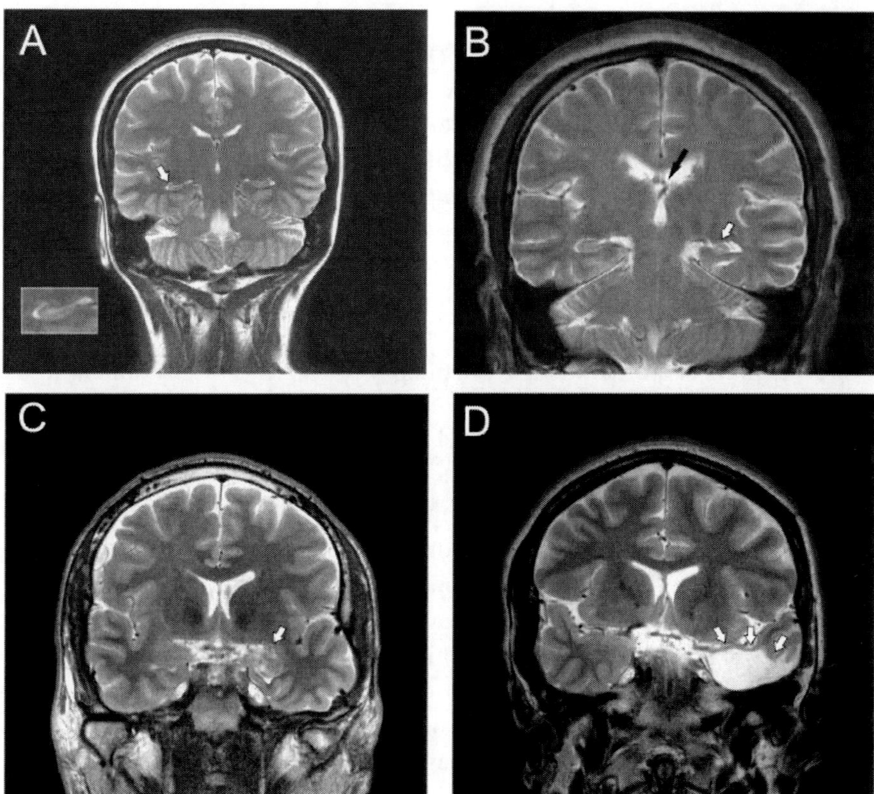

Figure 4. Four MRI images of the human brain showing epileptic damage to the limbic system. A, shows right hippocampal atrophy with mild signal hyperintensity (brightness), indicative of hippocampal sclerosis (white arrow). Note also the preserved delineation of Ammon's horn that is clearly seen on both sides, which is typical lost on the affected side in hippocampal sclerosis (see insert). B, shows dramatic left hippocampal atrophy (white arrow) as well as atrophy of the fornix on the left (black arrow). C, shows a multi cystic lesion of the left amygdala. The appearance is highly suggestive of a dysembryoplastic neuroepithelial tumor (DNET), which is often described as "tumor-like developmental lesion". There is often cortical dysplasia on the margins of the DNET proper, and it may be from this dysplastic tissue that the epiileptogenic tendency arises. D, shows what a typical anterior temporal resection looks like in the coronal plane. Note that the basal and inferior lateral temporal neocortex have been removed in order to gain access to the hippocampus. The lateral resection is extended back about 4-5 cm from the tip of the temporal lobe which gives the surgeon a window to resect all the way to the tail of the hippocampus.

Limbic System and Epilepsy

The limbic system is the origin of many seizures; limbic seizures (temporal lobe epilepsy, TLE, or medial temporal lobe epilepsy, MTLE) are mostly attributed to pathology in the hippocampus, such as the well described condition termed Ammon's horn sclerosis, in which many of the hippocampal principal cells have degenerated ([21-23]; Figure 4B). However, more recent studies have shown that the parahippocampal region may also play an important role ([24]; Figure 4C). This region sustains a characteristic pattern of damage in most animal models of epilepsy that is remarkably similar to that identified in humans with intractable temporal lobe epilepsy. Perhaps the most striking aspect of parahippocampal cortical pathology in epilepsy is the marked loss of neurons in layer III of the entorhinal cortex [25].

Partial-onset epilepsy arising in the temporal lobe has been associated with several types of pathologic lesions including Ammon's horn sclerosis, malformations, neoplasms, and inflammatory scars from infarcts or infection. These lesions are usually situated at various sites in the medial temporal lobe, so that one of the enigmas of attempting to understand the pathogenesis of TLE pertains to the clinical manifestation of a single epileptic disorder that is associated with dissimilar lesions at dissimilar sites. The analysis of extra-hippocampal temporal cortices with magnetic resonance, indeed, demonstrated that in patients with temporal lobe epilepsy the entorhinal cortex and the parahippocampal region can be markedly reduced in volume [26] even in the absence of a clear radiological pattern of mesial temporal sclerosis, typically associated with a selective hippocampal damage [27, 28]. The above findings suggest that changes in excitability and network interactions in the EC (and possibly in the PRC) may precede the involvement of the hippocampus proper during the development of temporal lobe epilepsy [24, 29].

Neurons in the neocortex have the capacity for plasticity, which is needed for is proper functioning, e.g., neuronal functioning in learning or in memory formation and storage [30, 31]. Neuronal plasticity emerges from a combination of the intrinsic function of the neurons within the circuit it is involved in, and the dynamics of circuit connectivity and function. However, the neural capacity for plasticity is accompanied by a significant risk: the capability to generate seizure discharges is also a property of all mammalian cortices. This leads to the fundamental question, how do cortical circuits reconcile the requirement to maintain plasticity, but at the same time control seizure initiation? This issue is especially important in the hippocampus since the hippocampus is a very plastic area in the brain due to its role in short-term memory formation, but is also a structure frequently implicated in the generation of epileptic seizures. For instance, temporal lobe epilepsy constitutes the most prevalent form of epilepsy in the adult population [32]. One aspect of hippocampal circuits that are particularly prominent are its intimate interconnections with the entorhinal cortex (Figure 3). These interconnections create a number of putative excitatory synaptic loops within this part of the limbic system leading to the possibility of reentrant activation and seizure generation in these loops. The hippocampus receives one primary cortical input: i.e., the perforant path, as mentioned above, innervates the dentate gyrus (DG), but a second input to the hippocampus also arises from the EC, the temporoammonic pathway (Figure), this pathway originates in layer III EC neurons and innervates the distal dendrites of area CA3 and CA1 in stratum lacunosum moleculare and subicular neurons in stratum radiatum [33]. The EC receives in turn hippocampal output axons, especially from the subiculum [34], therefore at least two primary excitatory loops exist. A long loop is created, incorporating the canonical hippocampal trisynaptic pathway (Figure) with the loop being closed via subiculum to EC; and an intermediate-length loop incorporates area CA3 (to CA1 to subiculum to EC); and finally, a shorter loop that involves direct EC input to area CA1 with the loop being closed via subiculum and EC. These pathways are summarized in the trisynaptic circuit diagram (Figure 3). Furthermore, especially in non-primate species, the left and right hippocampus are also interconnected [35, 36]. It is of interest to note that the reduction in hippocampal commissural connections is associated with the increase in laterality in brain functioning.

These excitatory synaptic loops in the hippocampus are important in normal hippocampal functioning, but also are involved in creating an underlying predisposition of the hippocampus and associated limbic structures to generate seizures [37, 38]. One hypothesis that has been posited is that, to regulate this vulnerability, both the dentate gyrus and area CA1 exhibit specialized properties i.e., interneuron circuits to make it less likely that excitatory inputs will escape control and trigger seizures (cf. [39]). The future careful study of the dynamics of circuit function will facilitate the characterization of these control mechanisms, allowing them to be compared and contrasted between structures, both in the normal brain and in the brains of epileptic animals at varying times during development of epilepsy.

The so-called "hippocampal sclerosis" typically demonstrates a pattern of preferential neuronal loss and astrogliosis both in CA4 (a.k.a end-folium area) and CA1 subfields more than in the CA3 subfield and granule cell layer of the dentate gyrus, and little to no neuronal loss in the CA2 subfield. In general, hippocampal sclerosis involves the selective loss of some excitatory hippocampal neuronal populations, in a process that likely will disturb the excitatory/inhibitory balance of the remaining cells and thereby could produce an epileptic focus. Sclerosis of the endfolium (dentate gyrus hilar region; Figures 2 and 4) is the minimal common pathological change found in epileptic patients with hippocampal damage [40]. This subtle lesion is characterized by extensive dentate hilar cell loss without a similarly severe loss of dentate granule cells or hippocampal pyramidal neurons. Endfolium sclerosis can be experimentally produced by focal electrical stimulation of dentate granule cell leading to seizure discharges in anesthetized rats (thereby avoiding generalized seizure activity and motor convulsions). With this model, dentate hilar neurons and CA3 pyramidal cells are selectively and irreversibly injured, replicating the pattern of human endfolium sclerosis, with hilar cell damage and survival of dentate granule cell layer GABA-containing basket cells. This results in permanent granule cell disinhibition and hyperexcitability. Excitatory deafferentation of GABAergic basket cells is probably secondary to the loss of hilar mossy cells that normally excite the GABA neurons, rendering these neurons dormant. We propose that endfolium sclerosis in humans represents a selective loss of intrinsically vulnerable dentate hilar cells that normally govern dentate granule cell excitability and that this process leads to epileptiform discharges.

The limbic/mesial temporal lobe epilepsy syndrome has been defined as a focal epilepsy, with the implication that there is a well defined focus of onset, traditionally centered around the hippocampus. The pathology of the hippocampus in this syndrome has been well described and a number of physiological abnormalities have been defined in this structure in animal models and humans with epilepsy. However, anatomical and physiological abnormalities have also been described in other limbic sites in this form of epilepsy. Previous studies have shown broadly synchronized or multifocal seizure onset within the limbic system of the animal models and human patients. We hypothesized that the epileptogenic circuit for the initiation of seizures was distributed throughout the limbic system with a possible central synchronizing process. In vitro studies showed that multiple limbic sites in epileptic animals (hippocampus, entorhinal cortex, piriform cortex and amygdala) have epileptiform changes with prolonged depolarizations and multiple superimposed action potentials.

In animal models of temporal lobe epilepsy, it is likely that the normal hippocampal circuit control mechanisms controlling pathological activity have been damaged or lost. How are the circuit dynamics of EC input regulation preserved or lost in the dentate gyrus and in area CA1 of animals with epilepsy? In these animals, it is known that the properties of inhibition are significantly altered. Both inhibitory synaptic function and GABAA receptor expression and function are altered in the dentate gyrus [42, 43] and area CA1 [44]. This compromise in inhibition is manifest at the level of GABA receptors, transmembrane chloride gradients [43, 44], and GABA neurotransmitter replenishment [45].

Since inhibition is a powerful regulator of entorhinal cortex neuroanal input processing in both these circuits, this would lead to the prediction that both circuits should be significantly compromised. However, it has been shown that predominantly CA1 processing of entorhinal cortex input is affected. There is a dramatic loss of CA1 neurons' ability to appropriately regulate EC inputs, with a 10- to 20-fold increase in TA pathway response measures [46]. However, regulation of EC inputs by dentate granule cells was largely unchanged [47]. This preserved gating function of the dentate gyrus may be due, at least in part, to the overexpression of synaptic GABAA receptors in dentate granule cells of epileptic animals, a possible compensatory cellular response to hyperactivity in the hippocampus [48].

Recent demonstrations of alterations in temporal lobe anatomy, e.g., malformations of the normal circuitry of the temporal lobe and foci of microdysgenesis, have given rise to the hypothesis that insults which occur during a critical period of brain development could alter the connections within the hippocampus and predispose it to increased excitability and the genesis of seizures. Such a hypothesis forces us to reconsider TLE in reference to risk factors that produce these anatomical changes or malformations. These malformations may range from a subtle alteration in the neurotransmitters of the dentate gyrus to large areas of cortical dysplasia or the hamartomatous neoplasms seen in TLE. A reevaluation of the neuroanatomical disruptions created by the various lesions may allow us to define a minimal optimal surgical resection for each lesion. Furthermore, the establishment of neurotransmitter deficits may lead to alternative pharmacologic therapies. With the development of better MRI imaging techniques we have the exciting opportunity to participate in the definition of the neuropathology of temporal lobe epilepsy [49].

Functional Problems in TLE

The impact of epilepsy is multifaceted and is quite extensive in its effects. Most fundementally, the unpredictable occurrence of seizures poses significant risk of falls and other forms of injury (e.g. burns, broken teeth, dislocation of joints), or even death from drowning, head trauma, motor vehicle accident, or hypoxia associated with prolonged seizures (status epilepticus). In addition to those risks, 1-3 per 1000 epilepsy patients per year will die of Sudden Unexpected Death in Epilepsy (SUDEP) [50, 51]. SUDEP is defined as unexpected, nontraumatic and nondrowning death in patients with epilepsy, with or without evidence for a seizure and excluding documented status epilepticus, in which no anatomical or toxicologic cause of death is apparent [52]. Furthermore, epilepsy may lead to, stigmatization and social exclusion and can have detrimental effects on an individual's confidence and self-esteem. Even seizures that occur as infrequently as once every six months will prevent a patient from sustaining legal driving privileges, which may make finding gainful employment difficult.

However, the burden of epilepsy extends beyond the effects of seizures themselves. In addition to the physical risks, epilepsy carries an increased risk of mental health comorbidities such as anxiety and depression beyond that which can be attributed to disability [53]. Depression in epilepsy has been shown to be strongly correlated with negative impacts on subjective health status and quality of life, and treatment of depression in epilepsy has been shown to improve quality of life, often more so than reduction in seizure frequency.

Antiepileptic drug (AED) treatment is commonly associated with neuropsychological side effects, which further impair patients' quality of life. While not always present, sedation and cognitive slowing are risks with multiple AEDs, and that risk increases when AEDs are used in combination for difficult to control epilepsy cases. Some AEDs have very specific neuropsychological side effects, such as topiramate, which is known to cause word finding difficulty [54], levetiracetam, which may cause aggression, irritability and mood changes [55], and perampanel, an AED recently approved in the U.S., which is known to cause hostility and even homicidal ideation at high doses [56].

Because the hippocampus is the single most common site of seizure onset in adults, memory difficulties are a particular concern among many individuals with epilepsy, especially those with seizures arising in the language-dominant hemisphere. These memory impairments frequently result in underachievement in the academic and professional arenas and often continue to worsen with time, especially in those with treatment resistant epilepsy. While temporal lobe surgery is the most effective treatment for drug resistant TLE, if the patient has good preoperative memory performance resection of the mesial temporal structures will very frequently result in a significant decline in memory performance [57], therefore assessment of the functional status of both the epileptic hippocampus and the contralateral hippocampus is essential. The intracarotid amobarbital tests (a.k.a. Wada test) has been the most commonly used method to assess hippocampal functional adequacy and reserve [58], though emerging data suggests that functional MRI may help to lateralize both language function and memory function non-invasively [59].

Conclusion

Performing temporal lobe epilepsy (TLE) surgery needs secure knowledge of the surgical anatomy [23, 60]. The functional anatomy has to be known because the temporal lobe plays a major role in language and memory. Also of paramount importance are the visual and auditory pathways; they are in close relationships with the temporal horn. They project to the occipital calcarine banks and the temporal operculum, respectively. The anatomical structures delineating the temporal horn have also to be well-recognized by the surgeon from inside the ventricle, namely: the hippocampus with its tiny fimbria bundle, the choroidal fissure and its velum with the attached choroid plexus. Since any TLE surgery also consists of disconnections, the surgery should try to avopid the uncinate fascicle, the (intertemporal) anterior commissure, the fornix, and more generally the ipsilateral limbic system.

Functional MRI can help to lateralize language and localize primary motor, somatosensory and language areas, and shows promise for predicting the effects of temporal lobe resection on memory. Tractography can visualize the main cerebral white matter tracts, thereby predicting and reducing surgery risk. Currently, displays of the optic radiation and pyramidal tracts are the most relevant for epilepsy surgery. Reliable integration of structural and functional data into surgical image-guidance systems is being pursued, and promises safer neurosurgery for epilepsy in the future.

References

[1] Dieckhofer K: A historical review of epilepsy. Special aspects of historical development on the etiopathology of the falling sickness and the various terms of the "falling evil" throughout the centuries. *History of medicine* 7(1-2), 43-48 (1976).

[2] Sommer W: Erkrankung des Ammonshornes als aetiologisches Moment der Epilepsie. *Arch Psychiatr Nervenkr 361–375.*, (1880).

[3] Willis T: Cerebri anatome., (1664).

[4] Broca P: Anatomie compareé des circonvolutions cérébrales: grand lobe limbique et la scissure limbique dans la série des mammifères. *Revue Anthropologie* 21, 384-498 (1878).

[5] Le Clark WE: The olfactory brain or so-called rhinencephalon. *The Medical journal of Australia* 2(21), 755-756 (1952).

[6] Kluver H: Brain mechanisms and behavior with special reference to the rhinencephalon. *The Journal-lancet* 72(12), 567-574 (1952).

[7] Papez JW: A proposed mechanism of emotion. *Arch. Neurol. Pscychiatry* 38, 725-743 (1937).

[8] Klüver HaB, P.C.: "Psychic blindness" and other symptoms following bilateral temporal lobectomy. *Am. J. Physiol.* 119, 254-284 (1937).

[9] Maclean PD: Some psychiatric implications of physiological studies on frontotemporal portion of limbic system (visceral brain). *Electroencephalography and clinical neurophysiology* 4(4), 407-418 (1952).

[10] Nauta WJH: *Expanding borders of the limbic system concept.* In: *Functional Neurosurgery.*, (Ed.^(Eds). Raven Press, New York 7-23 (1979).

[11] Kotter R, Meyer N: The limbic system: a review of its empirical foundation. *Behavioural brain research* 52(2), 105-127 (1992).

[12] Stephan H, Andy OJ: Quantitative Comparisons of Brain Structures from Insectivores to Primates. *American zoologist* 4, 59-74 (1964).

[13] Heimer L, Van Hoesen GW: The limbic lobe and its output channels: implications for emotional functions and adaptive behavior. *Neuroscience and biobehavioral reviews* 30(2), 126-147 (2006).

[14] Stephan H: Evolutionary trends in limbic structures. *Neuroscience and biobehavioral reviews* 7(3), 367-374 (1983).

[15] Insausti R, Tunon T, Sobreviela T, Insausti AM, Gonzalo LM: The human entorhinal cortex: a cytoarchitectonic analysis. *The Journal of comparative neurology* 355(2), 171-198 (1995).

[16] Mohedano-Moriano A, Martinez-Marcos A, Pro-Sistiaga P et al.: Convergence of unimodal and polymodal sensory input to the entorhinal cortex in the fascicularis monkey. *Neuroscience* 151(1), 255-271 (2008).

[17] Carlsen J, De Olmos J, Heimer L: Tracing of two-neuron pathways in the olfactory system by the aid of transneuronal degeneration: projections to the amygdaloid body and hippocampal formation. *The Journal of comparative neurology* 208(2), 196-208 (1982).

[18] Insausti R, Marcos P, Arroyo-Jimenez MM, Blaizot X, Martinez-Marcos A: Comparative aspects of the olfactory portion of the entorhinal cortex and its projection to the hippocampus in rodents, nonhuman primates, and the human brain. *Brain research bulletin* 57(3-4), 557-560 (2002).

[19] Agster KL, Burwell RD: Hippocampal and subicular efferents and afferents of the perirhinal, postrhinal, and entorhinal cortices of the rat. *Behavioural brain research* 254, 50-64 (2013).

[20] Fell J, Klaver P, Elger CE, Fernandez G: The interaction of rhinal cortex and hippocampus in human declarative memory formation. *Reviews in the neurosciences* 13(4), 299-312 (2002).

[21] Thom M: Hippocampal sclerosis: progress since Sommer. *Brain pathology* 19(4), 565-572 (2009).

[22] Worrell GA, Sencakova D, Jack CR, Flemming KD, Fulgham JR, So EL: Rapidly progressive hippocampal atrophy: evidence for a seizure-induced mechanism. *Neurology* 58(10), 1553-1556 (2002).

[23] Duncan JS: Imaging in the surgical treatment of epilepsy. *Nature reviews. Neurology* 6(10), 537-550 (2010).

[24] De Curtis M, Pare D: The rhinal cortices: a wall of inhibition between the neocortex and the hippocampus. *Progress in neurobiology* 74(2), 101-110 (2004).

[25] Schwarcz R, Eid T, Du F: Neurons in layer III of the entorhinal cortex. A role in epileptogenesis and epilepsy? *Annals of the New York Academy of Sciences* 911, 328-342 (2000).

[26] Bernasconi N, Andermann F, Arnold DL, Bernasconi A: Entorhinal cortex MRI assessment in temporal, extratemporal, and idiopathic generalized epilepsy. *Epilepsia* 44(8), 1070-1074 (2003).

[27] Sloviter RS: On the relationship between neuropathology and pathophysiology in the epileptic hippocampus of humans and experimental animals. *Hippocampus* 4(3), 250-253 (1994).

[28] Bernasconi N, Bernasconi A, Andermann F, Dubeau F, Feindel W, Reutens DC: Entorhinal cortex in temporal lobe epilepsy: a quantitative MRI study. *Neurology* 52(9), 1870-1876 (1999).

[29] Sloviter RS: The functional organization of the hippocampal dentate gyrus and its relevance to the pathogenesis of temporal lobe epilepsy. *Annals of neurology* 35(6), 640-654 (1994).

[30] Tononi G, Cirelli C: Sleep and the price of plasticity: from synaptic and cellular homeostasis to memory consolidation and integration. *Neuron* 81(1), 12-34 (2014).

[31] Butz M, Worgotter F, Van Ooyen A: Activity-dependent structural plasticity. *Brain research reviews* 60(2), 287-305 (2009).

[32] Berg AT, Testa FM, Levy SR, Shinnar S: The epidemiology of epilepsy. Past, present, and future. *Neurologic clinics* 14(2), 383-398 (1996).

[33] Van Groen T, Miettinen P, Kadish I: The entorhinal cortex of the mouse: organization of the projection to the hippocampal formation. *Hippocampus* 13(1), 133-149 (2003).

[34] Van Groen T, Lopes Da Silva FH: Organization of the reciprocal connections between the subiculum and the entorhinal cortex in the cat: II. An electrophysiological study. *The Journal of comparative neurology* 251(1), 111-120 (1986).

[35] Van Groen T, Wyss JM: Species differences in hippocampal commissural connections: studies in rat, guinea pig, rabbit, and cat. *The Journal of comparative neurology* 267(3), 322-334 (1988).

[36] Stringer JL, Lothman EW: Bilateral maximal dentate activation is critical for the appearance of an afterdischarge in the dentate gyrus. *Neuroscience* 46(2), 309-314 (1992).

[37] Jones RS, Heinemann UF, Lambert JD: The entorhinal cortex and generation of seizure activity: studies of normal synaptic transmission and epileptogenesis in vitro. *Epilepsy research. Supplement* 8, 173-180 (1992).

[38] Stringer JL, Lothman EW: Reverberatory seizure discharges in hippocampal-parahippocampal circuits. *Experimental neurology* 116(2), 198-203 (1992).

[39] Lothman EW, Stringer JL, Bertram EH: The dentate gyrus as a control point for seizures in the hippocampus and beyond. *Epilepsy research. Supplement* 7, 301-313 (1992).

[40] Sloviter RS: Hippocampal pathology and pathophysiology in temporal lobe epilepsy. *Neurologia* 11 Suppl 4, 29-32 (1996).

[41] Wozny C, Knopp A, Lehmann TN, Heinemann U, Behr J: The subiculum: a potential site of ictogenesis in human temporal lobe epilepsy. *Epilepsia* 46 Suppl 5, 17-21 (2005).

[42] Sloviter RS, Dean E, Sollas AL, Goodman JH: Apoptosis and necrosis induced in different hippocampal neuron populations by repetitive perforant path stimulation in the rat. *The Journal of comparative neurology* 366(3), 516-533 (1996).

[43] Pathak HR, Weissinger F, Terunuma M. et al.: Disrupted dentate granule cell chloride regulation enhances synaptic excitability during development of temporal lobe epilepsy. *The Journal of neuroscience : the official journal of the Society for Neuroscience* 27(51), 14012-14022 (2007).

[44] Schwarzer C, Tsunashima K, Wanzenbock C, Fuchs K, Sieghart W, Sperk G: GABA(A) receptor subunits in the rat hippocampus II: altered distribution in kainic acid-induced temporal lobe epilepsy. *Neuroscience* 80(4), 1001-1017 (1997).

[45] Ortinski PI, Dong J, Mungenast A. et al.: Selective induction of astrocytic gliosis generates deficits in neuronal inhibition. *Nature neuroscience* 13(5), 584-591 (2010).

[46] Wozny C, Gabriel S, Jandova K, Schulze K, Heinemann U, Behr J: Entorhinal cortex entrains epileptiform activity in CA1 in pilocarpine-treated rats. *Neurobiology of disease* 19(3), 451-460 (2005).

[47] Ang CW, Carlson GC, Coulter DA: Massive and specific dysregulation of direct cortical input to the hippocampus in temporal lobe epilepsy. *The Journal of neuroscience : the official journal of the Society for Neuroscience* 26(46), 11850-11856 (2006).

[48] Brooks-Kayal AR, Shumate MD, Jin H, Rikhter TY, Coulter DA: Selective changes in single cell GABA(A) receptor subunit expression and function in temporal lobe epilepsy. *Nature medicine* 4(10), 1166-1172 (1998).

[49] So EL: Role of neuroimaging in the management of seizure disorders. *Mayo Clinic proceedings* 77(11), 1251-1264 (2002).

[50] Ficker DM, So EL, Shen WK et al.: Population-based study of the incidence of sudden unexplained death in epilepsy. *Neurology* 51(5), 1270-1274 (1998).

[51] Opeskin K, Berkovic SF: Risk factors for sudden unexpected death in epilepsy: a controlled prospective study based on coroners cases. *Seizure: the journal of the British Epilepsy Association* 12(7), 456-464 (2003).

[52] Nashef L, So EL, Ryvlin P, Tomson T: Unifying the definitions of sudden unexpected death in epilepsy. *Epilepsia* 53(2), 227-233 (2012).

[53] Gilliam F, Kanner AM: Treatment of depressive disorders in epilepsy patients. *Epilepsy & behavior : E&B* 3(5S), 2-9 (2002).

[54] Mula M, Trimble MR, Thompson P, Sander JW: Topiramate and word-finding difficulties in patients with epilepsy. *Neurology* 60(7), 1104-1107 (2003).

[55] Bootsma HP, Ricker L, Diepman L. et al.: Long-term effects of levetiracetam and topiramate in clinical practice: A head-to-head comparison. *Seizure : the journal of the British Epilepsy Association* 17(1), 19-26 (2008).

[56] Steinhoff BJ, Ben-Menachem E, Ryvlin P. et al.: Efficacy and safety of adjunctive perampanel for the treatment of refractory partial seizures: a pooled analysis of three phase III studies. *Epilepsia* 54(8), 1481-1489 (2013).

[57] Hermann BP, Seidenberg M, Haltiner A, Wyler AR: Relationship of age at onset, chronologic age, and adequacy of preoperative performance to verbal memory change after anterior temporal lobectomy. *Epilepsia* 36(2), 137-145 (1995).

[58] Kneebone AC, Chelune GJ, Dinner DS, Naugle RI, Awad IA: Intracarotid amobarbital procedure as a predictor of material-specific memory change after anterior temporal lobectomy. *Epilepsia* 36(9), 857-865 (1995).

[59] Binder JR, Sabsevitz DS, Swanson SJ, Hammeke TA, Raghavan M, Mueller WM: Use of preoperative functional MRI to predict verbal memory decline after temporal lobe epilepsy surgery. *Epilepsia* 49(8), 1377-1394 (2008).

[60] Spencer DD, Spencer SS: Hippocampal resections and the use of human tissue in defining temporal lobe epilepsy syndromes. *Hippocampus* 4(3), 243-249 (1994).

In: The Limbic System
Editor: Russel T. Geary

ISBN: 978-1-63117-993-8
© 2014 Nova Science Publishers, Inc.

Chapter 2

The Limbic System and Chronic Musculoskeletal Pain

Kieran Macphail[*]
Bowskill Clinic, London, UK

Abstract

Emotions are often cited as a potential cause of musculoskeletal symptoms. However, the explanations given for this relationship are frequently vague and non-specific. This chapter focuses on the specific mechanisms by which the limbic system can influence musculoskeletal symptoms. A conceptual framework is presented suggesting conscious and sub conscious interpretation of emotional responses to events can impact all systems of the body generating or modifying musculoskeletal symptoms. The limbic system can directly modify the activity of the autonomic, endocrine, immune and musculoskeletal systems. Through these systems it is able to alter the activity of all other systems. In addition the limbic system is integral to our psychology which can similarly modify symptoms. It is important to note that multiple systems are being affected simultaneously. The end result may be that pain is felt in a specific region, which can be viewed within the context of current knowledge on pain physiology and the neuromatrix. An understanding of these processes may improve a clinician and patient's understanding of

---

[*] Corresponding author: Email: kieran@kieranmacphail.com.

what may be influencing symptoms. It is hoped this understanding may help improve outcomes.

Introduction

The link between how we cognitively process events and physical symptoms is often poorly described and abstract in its' thinking. However through an understanding of the limbic system clear pathways can be traced explaining some of these interactions. In reality this is a bidirectional relationship and needs to be viewed as part of an integrated web with many of these different pathways active simultaneously as part of the strive for homeostasis. This chapter focuses on how the limbic system can contribute to chronic musculoskeletal pain.

Pain can be viewed as a neurotag, an output of the neuromatrix and as an emotion regulated like temperature in order maintain homeostasis [1,2,3]. Nociception is neither sufficient nor necessary for the experience of pain [4,5]. The most widely accepted theory of pain is the neuromatrix [2]. Melzack's neuromatrix suggests that pain is an output and ultimately a conscious decision by the brain, based on the sum of all the inputs and past experience. From an evolutionary perspective a nociceptor's role is more than simply nociception but homeostasis [3].

The limbic system is integral to perception. The integration of past memories and experiences, with emotional context of the current input produces outputs that can modify the activity of the autonomic, endocrine, immune and musculoskeletal system. The hippocampus, amygdala and periaqueductal grey are of particular interest in this regard. The hippocampus is integral to long-term memory, which is important in terms of understanding the context of inputs, and has implications in the perception of events. The amygdala is important in these connections for its role in emotional motivation for behaviour and movement. As well as pain modulation, emotional responses to pain, and fear and reward related behaviours. The periaqueductal grey is not normally considered part of the limbic system but is functionally and neurally connected. The periaqueductal gray has important functions in pain modulation and defensive behaviour. Through these pathways the limbic system is able to indirectly influence all systems of the human body. Thus there are a plethora of mechanisms through which the limbic system can contribute to and modify musculoskeletal pain.

Autonomic Nervous System

The limbic system can produce an increase in sympathetic nervous system activity as a result of conscious and subconscious processing of inputs. In response to chronic stress the hypothalamic-pituitary-adrenal (HPA) axis initially goes in to hyper-function and over time this system becomes fatigued progressing to hypo-function [6]. This leads to a loss of negative feedback and a potentially pro-inflammatory situation. When done chronically this can contribute to musculoskeletal symptoms through several mechanisms such as exhausting the systems "raw materials", altering breathing mechanics, influencing skeletal and smooth muscle tone, reducing repair, increasing pain sensitivity and increasing stress reducing behaviours.

Prolonged increased sympathetic nervous system (SNS) stimulation leads to an increase requirement for the raw materials to run the fight or flight response eventually these resources can become depleted and exhausted which can contribute to musculoskeletal pain. For example chronic stress increases demands for minerals such as magnesium. If prolonged this can lead to a systemic deficiency, associated with symptoms such as trigger point formation and fibromyalgia [7].

Everybody has experienced the alterations in breathing pattern that occur when under perceived stress, but not everyone is aware of the impact these changes can have. Chaitow [8] outlined how breathing pattern disorders can contribute to the pain experience through biochemical, mechanical and nutritional mechanisms. Chronic hyperventilation can occur as a consequence of SNS hyperactivity. Low-level hyperventilation increases CO_2 losses, leading to a decrease in blood pH, otherwise known as a respiratory alkolosis. Nutritional effects occur as magnesium is "excreted" to increase pH, and loss of magnesium can assist in myofascial trigger point formation [9]. Myofascial trigger points are frequently associated with stress related musculoskeletal disorders such as fibromyalgia and myofascial pain syndrome. Additionally respiratory alkalosis leads to systemic vasoconstriction and muscles affected in this way are more prone to fatigue, thus less likely to be able to deal with imposed demands and more likely to become compromised.

Similarly most people have had the experience of being told to relax their shoulders and realising just how much tension they had been carrying. Empirically it is well established that increased SNS activity can increase muscle tone [10]. Importantly not all muscles are affected equally with the larger global muscles more suitable for running from predators most affected [11]. As joint stability relies on finely balanced muscle co-ordination between agonists and antagonists it is quite possible this could disrupt joint alignment and function predisposing to both acute and chronic injury [11]. Similarly, increased muscle tone increases compressive forces in joints, which at a threshold level may further contribute to symptoms. Smooth muscles cells are located in collagen within ligaments [12], intervertebral discs [13] and menisci [14]. These respond to sympathetic stimulation by contracting, as do the smooth muscle cells in arteries, which lead to vasoconstriction under periods of stress. From an evolutionary perspective this may have helped us be more biomechanically stable in fight or flight situations. However, as part of a chronic stress response this can contribute to the superficial tightness commonly seen in the clinic in patients with stress related musculoskeletal pain. These mechanical alterations of muscle tone and joint function may decrease the body's ability to deal with cumulative microtrauma.

Increased SNS activity impairs parasympathetic nervous system (PNS) activity, decreasing tissue repair and impairing the ability of the musculoskeletal system to handle cumulative microtrauma [15]. Chronic pain is multifaceted, the mechanical component can be viewed as a result of cumulative microtrauma and an inability of the body to sufficiently repair and adapt to the demands placed upon it. This concept suggests that an individual who runs excessively may have healthy knees at 90, whilst another with a healthier exercise routine may need both knees replaced at 60 due to insufficient tissue repair. If the 90 year old can sufficiently repair the tissues even with their excessive loading their knee may last well. However, if the 60 year old is very stressed, gets little sleep, and their parasympathetic system is hypoactive, then they may fail to repair their knee cartilage even with their comparatively low level demands.

Chronic psychological stress such as depression increases the sensation of the pain experience. For example depression is associated with a hyperactivity of the HPA axis and dysfunction of the serotonergic and noradrenergic systems [16]. These changes fundamentally increase the sensation of pain.

Some of the most common stress reducing behaviours are watching television, eating and drinking alcohol. One common theme from a health practitioner's perspective is that all these behaviours have a negative impact on musculoskeletal health. Alcoholism predates chronic pain and can arise after chronic pain. Furthermore, alcohol dependence and chronic pain share common circuits involving the amygdala. The reward and emotional circuits that regulate central sensation in chronic pain are also used for alcohol and drug dependence [17].

The stress response is perhaps the best understood mechanism through which the limbic system can influence the musculoskeletal system. The simple concept of running out of "raw materials" can be easy to explain to patients and may help to explain many common symptoms. Most of us are practically aware of the influence stress can have on our breathing pattern but the literature shows just how influential this often neglected compensation can be. The fairly linear process from stress to contraction of smooth muscle cells in fascia, and increased muscle tone is an easier concept for patients to grasp and most can relate to having experienced this. Through reducing repair and increasing pain intensity it is easy to see how many of the mechanisms will be working simultaneously. Confounding the effects of stress are the typically unhealthy ways individuals choose to manage stress, which often acerbate the negative effects on musculoskeletal health.

Endocrine System

The endocrine system is intimately related with the stress response through the HPA axis and the locus coeruleus. Chronic stress results in a hypoactive system characterised by reduced plasma levels of growth hormone and cortisol and is linked with fibromyalgia as well as other symptoms [18]. The sex hormone may also be influenced by the limbic system and can have marked effects on pain sensation and the musculoskeletal system.

The locus coeruleus noradrenergic system via the autonimic nervous system has systemic effects through the catecholamines epinephrine, norepinephrine and neuropeptide Y. The locus coeruleus noradrenergic system is consistently activated as a response to noxious stimuli [19]. Any input that threatens the biological, psychological or psychosocial integrity of the individual increases the firing rate of the locus coeruleus, increasing the turn over of norepinephrine [20]. Noradrenaline is excreted as a response to noxious stimuli and acts to suppress noccicpetion [21,22]. Patients with hypofunction of the sympathomedullary system may thus experience more pain. This assertion is supported by findings that patients with fibromyalgia have lower levels of noradrenaline metabolites.

Chronic stress leads to decreased plasma levels of growth hormone. The symptoms of growth hormone insufficiency such as fatigue and muscle weakness show similarities with those of fibromyalgia. Indeed approximately a third of fibromyalgia patients show signs of growth hormone deficiency [23], and sufferers show a decrease in spontaneous growth hormone secretion [24].

Suggesting a dysfunction at hypothalamic level in terms of neuroendocrine control of growth hormone. In the largest trial to date growth hormone treatment produced significantly reduced pain perception compared to placebo [25]. Thus the stress reaction mediated through the limbic system could play a role in chronic pain states through this mechanism.

Among the steroid hormones levels of oestrogens and testosterone are depleted in chronically stressed individuals. Elevated cortisol levels may lead to neuroendocrine dysfunction. Such dysfunction has been seen to decrease levels of oestrogens [26]. Oestrogens plays an essential role in bone turnover and thus this is a plausible mechanism for mechanical pain. Interestingly data from over 10,000 women who had hysterectomies and were randomly assigned to placebo or hormone replacement therapy, found that women treated with estradial were significantly less likely to have a joint replacement in the 7 years of the study [27].

There is currently no direct evidence levels of oestrogens can raise in response to limbic system activity. However, women exposed to pheromones from male armpits had increased length and timing of their menstrual cycles [28]. Another potential driver for excessive production of oestrogens is an increase in adipose tissue, which can contribute significantly circulating levels [29]. Thus indirectly through diet or behaviour it is possible the limbic system could contribute to elevated levels of oestrogens.

Oestrogens produce both pro- and antinociceptive effects and can modulate the nervous, immune, skeletal and cardiovascular systems [30]. Nonetheless there is considerable evidence oestrogens play a role in promoting migraine, temporomandibular dysfunction and fibromyalagia [31,32]. Furthermore females experience more pain than males to pressure, temperature, chemical stimuli and when focusing on the emotions associated with pain [33,34,35,36]. Additionally pain levels are generally higher when estradial levels peak [37]. Mechanically estradial stimulates the nucleus retroambiguus to cause an increase in lordosis in cats [38] and movement patterns alter during the menstrual cycle in response to hormonal changes [39]. Oestrogens may modify movement patterns as well as pain sensation contributing to musculoskeletal pain.

Testosterone levels are readily modified by exercise and diet, which are influenced by limbic system function. Other factors more directly influenced by the limbic such as self-esteem can also modify testosterone levels. For example fans of winning teams experience a rise in testosterone levels whereas supporters of loosing teams experience a drop in testosterone levels [40]. Similarly futures trader's testosterone levels rise on days they are successful and drop on days they are not [41]. Testosterone levels drop in men when they fall in love and rise in women, although these effects are transient [42]. Testosterone protects against TMJ pain in rats [43] and appears to decrease pain perception. In one study rats displayed significantly increased pain behaviour once castrated. However, the rat's behaviour normalised once testosterone therapy was administered [44].

The locus coeruleus noradrenergic system is stimulated by stress. Over time this can lead to hypo function and decreases in circulating levels of norepinephrine, testosterone and growth hormone, all of which help modulate the pain experience. Conversely oestrogens tend to promote nociception although there is limited evidence limbic activity can even indirectly increase oestrogen levels.

Immune System

The immune system response is an integral part of the pain experience and tissue healing. Lymphoid organs, cells, humoral factors and cytokines work independently with the endocrine and nervous systems to return the body to homeostasis [20]. Stress from many sources such as pain, relationships or depression can influence immune function. Mood has independently been associated with altered pain perception. The fast developing field of psychoneuroimmunology has helped elucidate some of the mechanisms for these interactions.

Psychoneuroimmunology has expanded on our understanding of neural and immune interactions. Pert et al. [45] found that neuropeptide receptors are present on the cell walls of both the brain and immune cells. Thus helping to explain the interaction between these systems. Many of the better-understood interactions in the brain-immune loop are mediated through the HPA axis though at this stage.

Stress and depression increase inflammation as does being in a troubled relationship. Similarly loneliness, sub clinical depression and major depression result in an increased inflammatory response to a stressful event. Stress and depression can also lead to obesity and adipose tissue further contributes pro-inflammatory cytokines. This can lead to a vicious cycle with depression contributing to inflammation and inflammation contributing to depression [46]. Specifically acute stress and major depression are associated with an increased leukocyte count and reduced natural killer cell counts, relative T-cell proportions, increases in CD4/CD8 ratios and decreases in T- and natural killer cell function. Random effects analysis suggested PGE2, IL-6 and circulating neutrophil levels would be higher in depression [47,48]. Chronic stress produces an increase in inflammation that may contribute to glucocorticoid resistance, which is associated with an increased local pro-inflammatory response [49]. It is suggested that patients with a more pro-inflammatory balance to their cytokines will be more likely to experience musculoskeletal symptoms.

Integrating these concepts, patients with pain 8 weeks after discectomy with greater sciatic pain were found to have elevated levels of IL-6, suffer from more depressed moods and have greater ongoing work related stress. Indeed the authors go as far as to suggest that ongoing sciatic pain may be associated with a relative adrenal and immune insufficiency [50]. This insufficiency leads to a lack of inhibition of pro-inflammatory mediators. This is an association and does not show any cause and effect. However, physiologically it's easy to see how it could.

The emerging field of psychoneuroimmunology has begun to elucidate some of the interactions in the brain-immune loop. The understanding of relationship between specific peptides and mood and immune effects is in its infancy, however our understanding of the HPA axis mediated effects of chronic stress and a pro-inflammatory cytokines is better established. It is suggested patients with a more systemic pro-inflammatory cytokine balance are more likely to experience musculoskeletal symptoms.

Musculoskeletal System

The motor system of the brain exists to translate thought, sensation, and emotion into movement. Thus allowing us to get what we need and communicate this to others both vocally and through body language [51]. Physical therapists have speculated that posture and movement disorders may be related to emotional states. Mood and anxiety have also been shown to effect postural control. None however have linked these to the pathways demonstrating the interaction of the limbic system on the motor system which has been mapped since the 1980s [52]. The limbic system has projections to the ventral tegmental area. The ventral tegmental area has projections to the nucleus accumbens and the nucleus accumbens has projections to the globus pallidus, which plays a key role in the regulation of voluntary movement. The emotional motor system (EMS) provides the circuitry for the translation of limbic system drives to movement.

headaches score higher on the Minnesota Multiphasic Personality Inventory, compared to patients with intracapsular temporomandibular joint disorders [62]. Type D or the "distressed personality", is especially sensitive to musculoskeletal symptoms. Mils et al. [63] compared the symptoms of cancer survivors with Type D personality with the remainder of 3080 subjects. 19% had Type D personality and they reported more back pain and osteoarthritis during the study. Similarly, in 5012 students aged 15-18, the 10.4% of boys and 14.6% of girls with Type D personality were twice as likely to have musculoskeletal pain, and five times more likely to have psychosomatic symptoms [64]. Furthermore in borderline personality disorder the key differences compared with controls on neuroimaging are found in the limbic system [65]. Specifically areas that control and regulate emotions show hypometabolism and limbic regions show hypermetabolism when activated. The amygdala in particular shows hypermetabolism in response to emotive images compared with controls.

The amygdala helps mediate the reciprocal relationship between chronic pain and negative affective states such as fear and anxiety. The amygdala has a known role in emotions and affective disorders, and it is now implicated in pain modulation and emotional responses to pain [66]. The lateral capsular division of the central nucleus of the amygdala is known as the nocciceptive amygdala, and appears to integrate internal and external environmental information with nocciceptive input. The amygdala can facilitate and inhibit pain at different levels of the pain neuraxis.

The "thought viruses" outlined by Butler and Moseley [1] highlight how the interactions between the hippocampus and amygdala can influence behviours that are associated with worse outcomes among chronic pain patients. Thoughts around the severity of symptoms and reducing activity to protect an area are all likely mediated at least partially through the limbic system. With memories of past advice and past experience retrieved from the hippocampus and the risk reward weighed up in the amygdala. These thoughts are known to be associated with withdrawing from normal activities and protecting painful areas of the body. This can lead to a lack of stress on connective tissues leading to atrophy, architectural disorganisation, fibrosis, adhesions and contractures. If inflammatory mediators are predominating then the tissue is more prone to fibrosis as opposed to atrophy [67]. Fibrosed and atrophied tissues are likely to lead to myofascial pain through differing mechanisms.

Taken a stage further, in some the pain experience will lead to receiving treatment or finding ways of managing the symptoms through altering posture.

Others receive encouragement to rest and possibly watch television in bed. Over time this behaviour is positively reinforced through operant conditioning and pain and behaviour may become learned [68]. This can lead to sickness behaviours and again is further associated with poorer outcomes.

An individual's psychology is an important factor influencing how people respond to musculoskeletal symptoms. A poor mood increases pain sensation. A type D personality is a significant consideration in patients with chronic pain, and is evidently associated with poor outcomes. The amygdala and hippocampus are integral to the circuitry that leads to "thought viruses" producing the protective behaviours linked with illness behaviour and worse symptomatology. These behaviours may become learned and reinforced leading to the downward spiral towards chronic pain.

Conclusion

This chapter has highlighted specific mechanisms through which the limbic system can contribute to chronic musculoskeletal pain. The stress response is mediated by perception, which is intimately related to the limbic system. Through the HPA axis the autonomic nervous system and endocrine system are able to exert powerful effects on the body, that can contribute to chronic musculoskeletal pain. This can occur through exhausting the systems "raw materials", altering breathing mechanics, increasing skeletal and smooth muscle tone, reducing repair, increasing pain sensitivity and increasing unhealthy stress-reducing behaviours. Chronic stress causes decreases in circulating levels of norepinephrine, testosterone and growth hormone, all of which help modulate the pain experience. Conversely oestrogens tend to promote nociception although there is limited evidence limbic activity can even indirectly increase oestrogen levels. Psychoneuroimmunology has helped us understand some of the impact of chronic stress on the HPA axis. Interestingly this stress can come from a variety of sources including pain, relationships or depression, and even mood can alter pain perception. From an evolutionary perspective the motor system exists to allow the limbic system to get what it wants and communicate this to others. The emotional motor system is the circuitry that allows this to take place. An individual's psychology is an important factor influencing how people respond to musculoskeletal symptoms. A Type D personality is a risk factor associated with worse outcomes. "Thought viruses" can produce protective behaviours linked with illness behaviour that may become learned and reinforced leading to downward spiral towards chronic pain. It is important to note that multiple systems are being affected simultaneously. Therapists should consider the limbic system's ability to modify and potentially chronic pain. An understanding of these processes may improve clinician and patient understanding of what may be influencing symptoms. It is hoped this understanding may help improve outcomes.

References

[1]   Butler, D. S. & Moseley, G. L. (2013). *Explain Pain*, (Revised and Updated. Noigroup Publications.

[2]   Melzack, R. (1999). From the gate to the neuromatrix. *Pain, 82,* S121-S126.

[3]   Craig, A. D. (2003). A new view of pain as a homeostatic emotion. *Trends in neurosciences, 26*(6), 303-307.

[4]   Puentedura, E. J. & Louw, A. (2012). A neuroscience approach to managing athletes with low back pain. *Physical Therapy in Sport, 13*(3), 123-133.

[5]   Acerra, N. E. & Moseley. (2005). Dysynchiria: watching the mirror image of the unaffected limb elicits pain on the affected side. *Neurology, 65*(5), 751-753.

[6]   Blackburn-Munro, G. & Blackburn-Munro, R. (2003). Pain in the brain: are hormones to blame?. *Trends in Endocrinology & Metabolism, 14*(1), 20-27.

[7]   Goldenberg, D. L. (1994). Fibromyalgia, chronic fatigue syndrome, and myofascial pain syndrome. *Current opinion in rheumatology, 6*(2), 223.

[8]   Chaitow, L. (2004). Breathing pattern disorders, motor control, and low back pain. *Journal of Osteopathic Medicine, 7*(1), 33-40.

[9]   Simons, D., Travell, J. & Simons, L. (1999) Myofascial pain and dysfunction: *the trigger point manual*, Vol *1*, upper half of body. (2nd ed.)Williams and Wilkins, Baltimore.

[10]   Needle, A. R., Baumeister, J., Kaminski, T. W., Higginson, J. S., Farquhar, W. B. & Swanik, C. B. (2014). Neuromechanical coupling in the regulation of muscle tone and joint stiffness. *Scandinavian Journal of Medicine & Science in Sports.*

[11]   Page, P., Frank, C. C. & Lardner, R. (2010). *Assessment and treatment of muscle imbalance: The Janda Approach*, Human Kinetics.

[12] Meiss, R. A. (1993). Persistent mechanical effects of decreasing length during isometric contraction of ovarian ligament smooth muscle. *J Muscle Res Cell Motil, 14*(2), 205-18.

[13] Hastreite, D. et al. (2001). Regional variations in certain cellular characteristics in human lumbar intervertebral discs, including the presence of -smooth muscle actin. *Journal of Orthopaedic Research, 19*(4), 597-604.

[14] Ahluwalia, S. (2001). Distribution of smooth muscle actin-containing cells in the human meniscus. *Journal of Orthopaedic Research, 19*(4), 659-664.

[15] Wallden, M. (2013). The primal nature of core function: In rehabilitation & performance conditioning. *Journal of bodywork and movement therapies, 17*(2), 239-248.

[16] Kandel, E. R. (2000). Disorders of Mood: Depression, Mania, and Anxiety Disorders. In: *Principles of Neural Science*. Eds. E.R. Kandel, J.H. Schwartz and T.M. Jessell. Mcgraw- Hill: New York. 1209-1226.

[17] Apkarian, A. V., Neugebauer, V., Koob, G., Edwards, S., Levine, J. D., Ferrari, L. & Regunathan, S. (2013). Neural mechanisms of pain and alcohol dependence. *Pharmacology Biochemistry and Behavior, 112*, 34-41.

[18] Lentjes, E. G. W. M. et al. (1997) Glucocorticoid receptors, fibromyalgiaand low back pain. *Psychoneuroendocrinology, 22*, 603–614.

[19] Svensson, T. H. (1987). Peripheral, autonomic regulation of locus coeruleus noradrenergic neurons in brain: putative implications for psychiatry and psychopharmacology. *Psychopharmacology, 92*, 1–7.

[20] Chapman, C. R., Tuckett, R. P. & Song, C. W. (2008). Pain and stress in a systems perspective: reciprocal neural, endocrine, and immune interactions. *The Journal of Pain, 9*(2), 122-145.

[21] Guo, T. Z., Jiang, J. Y., Buttermann, A. E. & Maze, M. (1996). Dexmedetomidine injection into the locus ceruleus produces antinociception, *Anesthesiology, 84*, 873-81.

[22] Pertovaara, A., Kauppila, T., Jyvasjarvi, E. & Kalso, E. (1991). Involvement of supraspinal and spinal segmental alpha-2-adrenergic mechanisms in the medetomidine-induced antinociception, *Neuroscience, 44*, 705-14.

[23] Cuatrecasas, G., González, M. J., Alegre, C., Sesmilo, G., Fernández-Solà, J., Casanueva, F. F., ... & Puig-Domingo, M. (2010). High prevalence of growth hormone deficiency in severe fibromyalgia

syndromes. *Journal of Clinical Endocrinology & Metabolism*, *95*(9), 4331-4337.

[24] Leal-Cerro, A. et al. (1999) The growth hormone (GH)-releasing hormone–GH–insulin-like growth factor-1 axis in patients with fibromyalgia syndrome. *J. Clin. Endocrinol. Metab.*, *84*, 3378–3381.

[25] Cuatrecasas, Guillem, et al. (2012). Growth hormone treatment for sustained pain reduction and improvement in quality of life in severe fibromyalgia. *Pain*, *153*(7), 1382-1389.

[26] Goldstein, J. M. (2006). Sex, hormones and affective arousal circuitry dysfunction in schizophrenia. *Hormones and behavior*, *50*(4), 612-622.

[27] Cirillo, D. J., Wallace, R. B., Wu, L. & Yood, R. A. (2006). Effects of hormone therapy on risk of hip and knee joint replacement in the *Women's Health Initiative Arthritis Rheum*, *54*, 3194–3204.

[28] Preti, G., Wysocki, C. J., Barnhart, K. T., Sondheimer, S. J. & Leyden, J. J. (2003). Male axillary extracts contain pheromones that affect pulsatile secretion of luteinizing hormone and mood in women recipients. *Biology of reproduction*, *68*(6), 2107-2113.

[29] Nelson, L. R. & Bulun, S. E. (2001). Estrogen production and action. *J Am Acad Dermatol*, *45*(3), S116-24.

[30] Craft, R. M. (2007). Modulation of pain by estrogens. *Pain*, *132*, S3-S12.

[31] Berkley, K. J. (1997). Sex differences in pain. *Behav. Brain Sci.*, *20*, 371–380

[32] Unruh, A. M. (1996). Gender variations in clinical pain experience. *Pain*, *65*, 123–167.

[33] Chesterton, L. S., Barlas, P., Foster, N. E., Baxter, G. D. & Wright, C. C. (2003). Gender differences in pressure pain threshold in healthy humans. *Pain*, *101*, 259–266.

[34] Sarlani, E., Farooq, N. & Greenspan, J. D. (2003). Gender and laterality differences in thermosensation throughout the perceptible range. *Pain*, *106*, 9–18.

[35] Frot, M., Feine, J. S. & Bushnell, M. C. (2004). Sex differences in pain perception and anxiety. A psychophysical study with topical capsaicin. *Pain*, *108*, 230–236.

[36] Keogh, E. & Herdenfeldt, M. (2002). Gender, coping and the perception of pain. *Pain 97*, 195–201.

[37] Fillingham, R. B. & Ness, T. J. (2000). Sex-related hormonal influences on pain and analgesic responses. *Neurosci. Biobehav. Rev.*, *24*, 485–501.

[38] De Greef, W. J., Schenck, P. E., Vreeburg, J. T. M., Van Der Vaart P. D. M. & Baum, M. J. (1981). Evidence that a placental factor other than androsterone or dihydrotestosterone inhibits oestrogen-induced lordosis behaviour in pregnant rats. *Journal of endocrinology, 89*, 13-23.

[39] Cesar, G. M., Pereira, V. S., Santiago, P. R. P., Benze, B. G., da Costa, P. H. L., Amorim, C. F. & Serrão, F. V. (2011). Variations in dynamic knee valgus and gluteus medius onset timing in non-athletic females related to hormonal changes during the menstrual cycle. *The Knee, 18*(4), 224-230.

[40] Bernhardt, P. C., Dabbs Jr, J. M., Fielden, J. A. & Lutter, C. D. (1998). Testosterone changes during vicarious experiences of winning and losing among fans at sporting events. *Physiology & Behavior, 65*(1), 59-62.

[41] Coates, J. M. & Herbert, J. (2008). Endogenous steroids and financial risk taking on a London trading floor. *Proceedings of the national academy of sciences, 105*(16), 6167-6172.

[42] Marazziti, D. & Canale, D. (2004). Hormonal changes when falling in love. *Psychoneuroendocrinology, 29*(7), 931-936.

[43] Fischer, L., Clemente, J. T. & Tambeli, C. H. (2007). The protective role of testosterone in the development of temporomandibular joint pain. *The Journal of Pain, 8*(5), 437-442.

[44] Pednekar, J. R. & Mulgaonker, V. K. (1995). Role of testosterone on pain threshold in rats. *Indian J Physiol Pharmacol, 39*(4), 423-4.

[45] Pert, C. B., Ruff, M. R., Weber, R. J. & Herkenham, M. (1985). Neuropeptides and their receptors: a psychosomatic network" *J Immunol, 135* (2), 820s-826s.

[46] Jaremka, L. M., Lindgren, M. E. & Kiecolt-Glaser, J. K. (2013). Synergistic relationships among stress, depression, and troubled relationships: insights from psychoneuroimmunology. *Depression and anxiety, 30*(4), 288-296.

[47] Zorrilla, E. P., Luborsky, L., McKay, J. R., Rosenthal, R., Houldin, A., Tax, A. & Schmidt, K. (2001). The relationship of depression and stressors to immunological assays: a meta-analytic review. *Brain, behavior, and immunity, 15*(3), 199-226.

[48] Ader, R., Cohen, N. & Felten, D. (1995). Psychoneuroimmunology: interactions between the nervous system and the immune system. *The Lancet, 345*(8942), 99-103.

[49] Cohen, S., Janicki-Deverts, D., Doyle, W. J., Miller, G. E., Frank, E., Rabin, B. S. & Turner, R. B. (2012). Chronic stress, glucocorticoid

receptor resistance, inflammation, and disease risk. *Proceedings of the National Academy of Sciences, 109*(16), 5995-5999.

[50] Geiss, A., Varadi, E., Steinbach, K., Bauer, H. W. & Anton, F. (1997). Psychoneuroimmunological correlates of persisting sciatic pain in patients who underwent discectomy. *Neuroscience Letters, 237*(2), 65-68.

[51] De Gelder, B. (2006). Towards the neurobiology of emotional body language. *Nature Reviews Neuroscience, 7*(3), 242-249.

[52] Mogenson, G. J., Jones, D. L. & Yim, C. Y. (1980). From motivation to action: functional interface between the limbic system and the motor system. *Progress in neurobiology, 14*(2), 69-97.

[53] Denys-Struyf, G. (2010). La structuration psychocorporelle de l'enfant. La vague de croissance selon la méthode G.D.S – ICTGDS – Bruxelles.

[54] Bolmont, B., Gangloff, P., Vouriot, A. & Perrin, P. P. (2002). Mood states and anxiety influence abilities to maintain balance control in healthy human subjects. *Neuroscience letters, 329*, 96–100.

[55] Wada, M., Sunaga, N. & Nagai, M. (2001). Anxiety affects the postural sway of the antero-posterior axis in college students, *Neuroscience letters, 302*, 157–159.

[56] Holstege, G. (1997). The emotional motor system. In: *The Encyclopedia of Human Biology, 3*, 2nd ed. Academic Press, San Diego, 643–660.

[57] Lovick, T. A. (1996). Midbrain and medullary regulation of defensive cardiovascular functions. *Progressive brain research, 107*, 301–313.

[58] Holstege, G. (1998a). The emotional motor system in relation to the supraspinal control of micturition and mating behavior. *Behavioural Brain Research, 92* (2), 103-109.

[59] Holstege, G. (1998b). The Anatomy of the Central Control of Posture: Consistency and Plasticity. *Neuroscience and biobehavioral reviews, 22* (4), 485-493.

[60] Zelman, D. C., Howland, E. W., Nichols, S. N. & Cleeland, C. S. (1991). The effects of induced mood on laboratory pain. *Pain, 46*(1), 105-111.

[61] McFadden, I. J. & Woitalla, V. F. (1993). Differing reports of pain perception by different personalities in a patient with chronic pain and multiple personality disorder. *Pain, 55*(3), 379-382.

[62] Mongini, F., Ciccone, G. & Ibertis, F. (2000). Personality characteristics and accompanying symptoms in temporomandibular joint dysfunction, headache, and facial pain. *Journal of orofacial Pain, 14*(1).

[63] Mols, F., Oerlemans, S., Denollet, J., Roukema, J. A. & van de Poll-Franse, L. V. (2012). Type D personality is associated with increased

comorbidity burden and health care utilization among 3080 cancer survivors. *General hospital psychiatry, 34*(4), 352-359.

[64] Condén, E., Leppert, J., Ekselius, L. & Åslund, C. (2013). Type D personality is a risk factor for psychosomatic symptoms and musculoskeletal pain among adolescents: a cross-sectional study of a large population-based cohort of Swedish adolescents. *BMC pediatrics, 13*(1), 11.

[65] Lis, E., Greenfield, B., Henry, M., Guilé, J. M. & Dougherty, G. (2007). Neuroimaging and genetics of borderline personality disorder: a review. *Journal of psychiatry & neuroscience, 32*(3), 162.

[66] Neugebauer, V., Li, W., Bird, G. C. & Han, J. S. (2004). The amygdala and persistent pain. *The Neuroscientist, 10*(3), 221-234.

[67] Langevin, H. M. & Sherman, K. J. (2007). Pathophysiological model for chronic low back pain integrating connective tissue and nervous system mechanisms. *Medical hypotheses, 68*(1), 74-80.

[68] Tyrer, S. P. (1986). Learned pain behaviour. *British medical journal (Clinical research ed.), 292*(6512), 1.

In: The Limbic System
Editor: Russel T. Geary

ISBN: 978-1-63117-993-8
© 2014 Nova Science Publishers, Inc.

Chapter 3

The Effects of Altered Gravity on the Limbic System

Robert Lalonde[1] and Catherine Strazielle[2]*

[1]R. Lalonde, Université de Rouen, Dépt. Psychologie, Laboratoire ICONES EA 4699, Mont-Saint-Aignan Cedex France
[2]Université de Lorraine, Laboratoire Stress, Immunité, Pathogènes EA 7300, and Service de Microscopie Electronique, Faculté de Médecine, Vandœuvre-les-Nancy, France, CHU de Nancy, Vandoeuvre-les-Nancy, France

Abstract

Changes in gravity conditions have often been shown to affect vestibulo-cerebellar functioning. In the present review, we describe recent experiments indicating a role for hypogravity and hypergravity on limbic system functioning. The effects of spaceflight on the limbic system include changes in cell diameter and monoamine levels as well as immediate early gene products. A method to determine the effects of hypogravity while earthbound is the hindlimb unloading response in rodents. Like spaceflight, hindlimb unloading causes changes in neuropeptide levels and cell stress responses. To gauge the complete actions of gravity changes, hypergravity induced by acceleration of caged but freely moving rodents placed inside a centrifuge has been examined.

[*] Corresponding author: Tel: +33 02 35 14 61 08, Fax: +33 02 35 14 63 49, Email: robert.lalonde@univ-rouen.fr.

Notable changes include altered mRNA levels of several genes expressed in the hippocampus. These results are discussed in the context of interactions between vestibulo-cerebellar areas and the limbic system under changes in gravity conditions.

1. Anatomical Relations between Vestibulocerebellum and the Limbic System

The effects of gravity on the brain have mostly been examined at the sensorimotor level, especially the vestibular system, since gravity receptors for linear acceleration in the otolith organs (utricule and saccule for horizontal and vertical movements, respectively) are unloaded in microgravity and overloaded in hypergravity (Bruce, 2003). Central vestibulospinal pathways include the limbic system (Goldberg et al., 2012). Effects on the limbic system may be mediated by vestibular neurons projecting via multisynaptic inputs to the hippocampus (Stackman et al., 2002). Indeed, vestibular lesions cause neurochemical or electrophysiologic alterations in the hippocampus (Besnard et al., 2012; Smith et al., 2005; Tai and Leung, 2012). Intermediary structures may comprise dorsal tegmental, lateral mammillary, and anterior thalamic nuclei, or pedunculopontine, supramamillary, and medial septal nuclei (Smith et al., 2005). In particular, the hippocampus depends on vestibular input to establish accurate spatial representations (Smith and Zheng, 2013), liable to deteriorate in rodents under conditions of hypogravity (Temple et al., 2002) or hypergravity (Feng et al., 2010; Francia et al., 2004; Mandillo et al., 2003; Mitani et al., 2004). Sometimes, vestibular (Douglas et al., 1979; Machado et al., 2012) lesions mimic hippocampal (Kirkby et al., 1967; Roberts et al., 1962) ones in spatial tests such as spontaneous alternation (Lalonde, 2002). Changes in gravity may also affect the limbic system via glucocorticoid receptors on hippocampal neurons responsible for negative feedback on blood corticosterone, the main hormone involved in stress reactions (Herman et al., 1989). The vestibular system may also influence the amygdala via the lateral parabrachial nucleus. The central nucleus of the amygdala receives and sends projections from and to the nucleus of the solitary tract either directly or indirectly via the lateral parabrachial nucleus (Ricardo and Koh, 1978; Saper and Loewy, 1980).

Vestibular nuclei are directly interconnected with the cerebellar cortex and the fastigial nucleus (Vidal and Sans, 2004). Electrophysiological evidence points towards indirect ascending fastigial projections to hippocampus, septum, and amygdala in the rat (Heath et al., 1978; Snider and Maiti, 1976). Other projections of relevance for the limbic system include those from cerebellar nuclei to the ventral midbrain tegmentum in the rat (Perciavalle et al., 1989; Snider et al., 1976). The fastigial nucleus of the cerebellum also influences neuroendocrine cells via the hypothalamus (Katafuchi et al., 1995). Indeed, electrophysiological evidence exists of direct connections between fastigial and paraventricular nuclei of the hypothalamus (Katafuchi and Koizumi, 1990). Head-down-tilt by tail suspension changed unit activity of the paraventricular nucleus of the hypothalamus, mostly by decreased firing rates, presumably because of information arising from baroreceptors in the thoracic activity, proprioceptors, and/or the vestibular organ (Katafuchi et al., 1987). Such vestibular influences are mediated via the fastigial nucleus because fastigial neurons respond to head-tilting (Ghelarducci, 1973).

The paraventricular nucleus of the hypothalamus is responsible for activating adrenocorticotropin from the anterior pituitary gland by releasing corticotropin-releasing hormone, thereby increasing corticosterone secretion from the adrenal cortex (Antoni, 1986). The paraventricular nucleus of the hypothalamus receives afferents from amygdala and septum (Armstrong, 2004; Palkovitz, 1986). Appetite and energy expenditure depend on the arcuate and ventromedial nuclei of the hypothalamus. The arcuate nucleus receives input from medial amygdala and lateral septum and the ventromedial nucleus from amygdala and ventral subiculum (Simerly, 2004).

2. Hypogravity and the Limbic System

2.1. Spaceflight

Spaceflight causes widespread changes in physiology, such as the regulation of extracellular fluid (Gauer et al., 1970) and muscle volume (Akima et al., 200)]. In Cosmos biosatellite flights lasting three weeks, there were metabolic and hormonal changes indicative of a moderate degree of stress without any pathological change in internal organs (Gazenko et al., 1980). Particular muscle groups were atrophied and their contractile properties adaptively transformed. Osteoporosis occurred and bone tissue decreased in durability. At the level of the brain, astronauts displayed changes in vestibular-related postural and eye movements, as well as spontaneous and reflex control of cardiovascular, respiratory, and gastrointestinal functions, sometimes associated with space motion sickness. All these symptoms underwent habituation over time. Da Silva et al. (2002) proposed that alterations of neuroendocrine mediators coordinating the stress response, mainly corticotropin-releasing hormone, is involved in the decreased appetite found during spaceflight. The effects of spaceflight were exerted as well in regard to oxidation mechanisms as indicated by interleukin-6 levels (Stein and Schluter, 1994).

2.1.1. Hypothalamus

The effects of spaceflight on the limbic system are summarized in Table 1. Mice that flew aboard the Apollo XVII vehicle had lower body weight than controls (Ordy et al., 1975). When hypothalamic morphology was examined, the nuclear diameter of supraoptic neurons responsible for secreting vasopressin was greater in flight mice than controls, a result not found in regard to the nuclear diameter in arcuate and ventromedial hypothalamic nuclei involved in appetite and energy expenditure. In rats aboard Cosmos 1129, concentrations of 5-hydroxytryptamine (5HT, serotonin) increased in the supraoptic nucleus but decreased in the periventricular nucleus (also involved in vasopressin release) and was unchanged in other hypothalamic nuclei (Culman et al., 1985). As a possible result, vasopressin content decreased in the hypothalamus of flight rats but increased in the posterior pituitary (Fareh et al., 1993). Nevertheless, Culman et al. (1985) concluded that long-term space flight does not represent a major stress factor with respect to 5HT in the hypothalamus.

Catecholamine levels in the hypothalamus were examined in rats aboard Soviet biosatellites of the Cosmos type (Kvetnansky et al., 1983). No change occurred in noradrenaline concentrations and in the activity of its synthesizing enzymes, tyrosine hydroxylase and dopamine-beta-hydroxylase, or its degrading enzyme, monoamine oxidase. However, when subnuclei of the hypothalamus were examined in rats aboard the Cosmos 1129 vehicle, noradrenaline levels diminished in arcuate and periventricular nuclei as well as the median eminence connecting the hypothalamus with the pituitary, and adrenaline levels diminished in periventricular and suprachiasmatic nuclei along with the median eminence. Moreover, noradrenaline content decreased in the locus coeruleus, site of origin of noradrenergic fibers to the forebrain (Fareh et al., 1994).

Table 1. Effects of spaceflight on the limbic system

Measures	Brain regions	Species	References
↑ neuron diameter	supraoptic nucleus of hypothalamus	mice	Ordy et al.,1975
↑ 5HT	supraoptic nucleus of hypothalamus	rats	Culman et al., 1985
↓ 5HT	periventricular nucleus of hypothalamus	rats	Culman et al., 1985
↓ noradrenaline	arcuate and periventricular nuclei of hypothalamus, locus coeruleus	rats	Fareh et al., 1994; Kvetnansky et al., 1983
↓ vasopressin	hypothalamus	rats	Fareh et al., 1993
↓ GFAP mRNA	hippocampus	rats	Day et al., 1998
↑ Fos	central nucleus of amygdala, locus coeruleus	rats	Centini and Pompeiano, 2007
↑ FRA	central nucleus of amygdala, locus coeruleus, hippocampus	rats	Centini and Pompeiano, 2007

2.1.2. Amygdala and Hippocampus

The amygdala is crucially involved in emotion, particularly fear responses, and the hippocampus in spatial orientation, functions liable to be modified during spaceflight. Mechanisms of cell stress have been examined in the hippocampus. A molecule of major interest in cell stress is glial fibrillary acidic protein (GFAP), highly expressed in glial cells. GFAP mRNA decreased in hippocampal subregions of rats exposed to spaceflight (Day et al., 1998). It was proposed that this effect is mediated by the increased serum corticosterone levels found in these rats, acting on hippocampal glucocorticoid receptors.

Pompeiano et al. (2004) proposed that short- and long-lasting molecular changes in medullary and basal forebrain gene expression play an important role in integrating autonomic and vestibular signals ultimately regulating neural adaptations to space flight. Several limbic regions were examined for immediate early gene products, Fos and Fos-related antigens (FRA) in flight rats killed at reentry and two weeks afterwards (Centini and Pompeiano, 2007). Fos and FRA are transcription factors regulating other genes (Herdegen and Leah, 1998). At reentry, Fos expression was higher than controls in central nucleus of the amygdala and locus coeruleus, but this was not so two weeks after landing. Also at reentry, FRA expression increased in locus coeruleus and nucleus paragigantocellularis lateralis of the medulla, the latter sending glutamatergic afferents to the locus coeruleus, as well as to structures producing corticotropin-releasing hormone, which activates noradrenergic neurons during stress. FRA expression also increased in the hippocampus and regions involved in EEG desynchronization and theta activity responsible for rapid eye movement (REM) sleep (Centini and Pompeiano, 2007). Likewise, FRA expression increased in the amygdaloid complex, particularly the central nucleus, as well as related structures such as the lateral parabrachial nucleus and the nucleus of the solitary tract. These regions contribute to pontine-geniculo-occipital (PGO) waves driving the oculomotor system either directly or through the medial vestibular nuclei. Such experiments provide molecular evidence that sources producing rhythmic discharges of vestibulo-ocular neurons during REM sleep may substitute for labyrinthine signals after exposure to microgravity, thus contributing to activity-related plastic changes and readaptation to normal gravity (Pompeiano, 2007).

2.2. Hindlimb Unloading

In addition to changes in gravity, spaceflight exposes astronauts to fluctuations in temperature, ultraviolet radiation, and other environmental contingencies. Antiorthostatic hindlimb unloading in rodents provides a method for determining the selective impact of hypogravity. In this experimental model, the tails of mice or rats are held by a restraining device so that the hindlimbs never touch ground and the head is tilted downward. Hindlimb unloading-induced hypogravity alters the vestibular system and proprioceptive muscle receptors which in turn affect selective brain regions. In particular, altered proprioceptive input from muscle receptors during tail suspension may be responsible for decreased gamma-aminobutyric acid (GABA) immunoreactivity found at axosomatic terminals in the pyramidal layer of rat somatosensory cortex (D'Amelio et al., 1998). Hindlimb unloading led to altered expression of over 500 genes when the whole brain was examined (Frigeri et al., 2008).

Hindlimb unloading is meant to test microgravity as such but should not always be expected to cause the same effects as spaceflight, because in addition to hypogravity up in space, hypergravity prevails at launch and landing (Morey-Holton and Globus, 2002). Unlike rats aboard SLS-1, hindlimb suspension did not decrease noradrenaline content in the locus coeruleus (Fareh et al., 1994). These results demonstrate that hindlimb-suspended rats sometimes adapt better to weightlessness-simulation than flight rats. The effects of hindlimb suspension are summarized in Table 2.

2.2.1. Hypothalamus

Like rats flown aboard SLS-1, hindlimb-suspended rats had lower vasopressin content in the hypothalamus (Fareh et al., 1994). Da Silva et al. (2002) reviewed the impact of the tail-suspension technique to mimic anorexia-related stress responses and proposed a role for corticotropin-releasing hormone and 5HT on microgravity-related decreases in food intake, delay in gastric emptying, and alterations of circadian rhythms. The acute impact of hindlimb suspension was examined on hypothalamic neuropeptides involved in appetite and energy expenditure in wild-type and *agouti* mice without access to food, the latter characterized by obesity and ectopic expression of the agouti protein, an antagonist of the melanocortin-4 receptor (Lew et al., 2009). Tail suspension for 3 hours increased oxygen consumption as well as carbon dioxide and heat production in wild-type mice and decreased their body weight. The increases in energy expenditure were not attenuated in agouti mice. Although tail suspension increased hypothalamic interleukin-6 mRNA levels in both groups, it did not alter mRNA levels of agouti-related protein, pro-opiomelanocortin (POMC), neuropeptide Y, or melanin concentrating hormone (MCH). These data support the hypothesis that short-term microgravity exposure increases energy expenditure via hypothalamic signaling pathways dependent on interleukin-6 but not necessarily melanocortins.

Table 2. Effects of hindlimb suspension on the limbic system

Measures	Brain regions	Species	References
↓ vasopressin	hypothalamus	rats	Fareh et al., 1994
↑ interleukin-6 mRNA	hypothalamus	mice	Lew et al., 2009
↓ glutathione	hypothalamus	mice	Sarkar et al., 2008
↑ nuclear transcription factor-kappaB, mitogen-activated protein kinase	hippocampus	mice	Wise et al., 2005
↓ pyruvate dehydrogenase	hippocampus	mice	Sarkar et al., 2008

Other molecules representing cell stress responses have been examined. Hindlimb suspension decreased glutathione levels in mouse hypothalamus (Sarkar et al., 2008). Proteomic analyses by gel electrophoresis revealed lower superoxide dismutase-2 as well as higher malate dehydrogenase and peroxiredoxin-6 in this brain region. These results indicate that hindlimb-suspended mice are vulnerable to pro-oxidant mechanisms and lead to the generation of reactive oxygen species.

2.2.2. Hippocampus

In addition to the hypothalamus, hindlimb suspension increased pro-oxidant mechanisms in the hippocampus as detected by activation of nuclear transcription factor-kappaB and mitogen-activated protein kinase (MAPK) as well as increased lipid peroxidation measured by levels of thiobarbiturate-reactive malondialdehyde (Wise et al., 2005). In addition, hindlimb suspension decreased pyruvate dehydrogenase expression in mouse hippocampus (Sarkar et al., 2008). This was probably not caused by general stress-mediated processes, because serum corticosterone levels were normal in these mice.

3. Hypergravity

To gauge the complete actions of gravity changes, researchers have assessed hypergravity induced by acceleration of caged but freely moving rodents, more rarely normal human subjects, placed inside a centrifuge. The effects of hypergravity on limbic regions are summarized in Table 3. Normal human subjects exposed to three times the normal force of gravity (3G) have altered electroencephalogram activities in the limbic lobe as indicated by increased beta-2 activity and decreased alpha-1 and beta-1 activities (Schneider et al., 2009). Hypergravity can alter at least on a short-term basis the circadian rhythms of mice and reduce their body mass via vestibular receptors (Fuller et al., 2004). Indeed, when *Nox3[het]* (*head-tilt*) mice mutated for NADPH oxidase 3 and lacking otoconia (macular gravity receptors) were compared to non-mutated mice, centrifugation at 2G altered circadian rhythms as well as decreased body mass and food intake in wild-type though to a lesser extent in mutant mice. The physiological impact of hypergravity is often caused by motion sickness, as gauged by the tendency of rodents to eat a non-nutritive substance, kaolin (pica behavior), an effect mitigated after bilateral labyrinthectomy (Sato et al., 2009; Uno et al., 1997).

3.1. Hypothalamus

After exposure to a centrifuge-induced 2G load, histamine release from the hypothalamus increased in rats along with kaolin consumption (Uno et al., 1997). These effects were not found after bilateral labyrinthectomy or after treatment with alpha-fluoromethylhistidine, an inhibitor of the histamine-synthesizing enzyme. Also during exposure to a 2G load in rats, mRNA expression of *Hrh1* encoding the H1 histamine receptor was up-regulated in the hypothalamus (Sato et al., 2009). The hypergravity-induced increase in kaolin intake was suppressed by mepyramine but not terfinadine or zolantizine, indicating that central but not peripheral postsynaptic H1 receptors or H2 receptors played a role in motion sickness.

Short- or long-term exposure to a 2G load induced Fos expression in arcuate and paraventricular nuclei of the hypothalamus and elevated the nociceptive threshold on rat skin surfaces concomitantly with evoked neuronal activity in the hypothalamus (Kumei et al., 2000, 2001, 2002). Fos expression was also induced in vestibular-related brainstem regions of rats exposed to a 2G load, as well as the entorhinal cortex (Gustave Dit Duflo et al., 2000), which indicate a possible interaction between the two regions.

Table 3. Effects of hypergravity induced by centrifugation on the limbic system

Measures	Brain regions	Species	References
↑ histamine release	hypothalamus	rats	Uno et al., 1997
↑ *Hrh1* mRNA	hypothalamus	rats	Sato et al., 2009
↑ Fos	arcuate and paraventricular nuclei of hypothalamus	rats	Kumei et al., 2000, 2001
↑ Fos	entorhinal cortex	rats	Gustave Dit Duflo et al., 2000
↓ Fos-positive neurons to light	suprachiasmatic nucleus of hypothalamus	rats	Murakami et al., 1998
↑ Fos	amygdala	rats	Nakagawa et al., 2003
↑ *Tac1* mRNA	amygdala	rats	Horii et al., 2012
↑ *Pcsk1n*	hippocampus	rats	Del Signore et al., 2004
↑ LTP	hippocampus	mice	Ishii et al., 2004
↑ GluR1 phosphorylation	hippocampus	mice	Ishii et al., 2004
↑ caspase-3 activity	hippocampus	rats	Feng et al., 2010

Murakami et al. (1998) examined the effect of hypergravity on the retinohypothalamic tract. Rats were exposed to 2 or 21 days of 2G centrifugation. During the last hour of 2G exposure, one series of rats was exposed to a 1 hour phase-shifting light pulse while the second was not. The controls showed the normal response to light when greater numbers of Fos-positive neurons were found in the suprachiasmatic nucleus of light-pulsed rats relative to that of nonlight-pulsed rats. However, rats exposed for 2 days to 2G did not show the same response to light. A recovery in the effect of light to induce Fos reactivity occurred in rats exposed to 21 days of 2G. These results indicate that exposure to 2G temporarily suppressed the responsiveness of the nucleus to the phase-shifting effects of light mediated by the retinohypothalamic tract.

3.2. Amygdala

A 2G load increased the number of Fos-expressing cells in the central nucleus of the amygdala together with vestibular nuclei, indicating the probable influence of changed vestibular input on neural activity in the limbic system (Nakagawa et al., 2003). The mRNA expression of *Tac1* (preprotachykinin 1, neurokinin-1 or substance P) and its receptor *Tacr1* (tachykinin receptor 1, or neurokinin receptor 1) was measured in the basolateral amygdala and the nucleus of the solitary tract after a 2G load in rats (Horii et al., 2012). *Tac1* mRNA expression increased in both regions, whereas *Tacr1* mRNA expression was unchanged. Nevertheless, a tachykinin receptor-1 antagonist mitigated motion sickness estimated by kaolin consumption in a dose-dependent and enantioselective manner. Hypergravity-induced motion sickness in rats measured by pica behavior also decreased after bilateral lesions of the amygdala (Uno et al., 2000).

3.3. Hippocampus

The effects of hypergravity on the hippocampus have been examined in view of its crucial importance in spatial learning, liable to deteriorate under conditions of hypergravity (Feng et al., 2010; Temple et al., 2002). In addition, the hippocampus plays a role in appetite (Tracy et al., 2001), also liable to be modified after a period of hypergravity (Lew et al., 2009). These effects are possibly mediated by glucocorticoid receptors in the hippocampus (Herman et al., 1989). Indeed, glucocorticoid hippocampal receptors have been shown to play a role in spatial learning (Bodnoff et al., 1995; de Quervain et al., 1998; Roozendaal et al., 2003).

Exposure to a 2G load altered mRNA levels of several genes expressed in the hippocampus, including *Pcsk1n*, encoding proprotein convertase subtilisin/kexin type 1 inhibitor (granin-like neuroendocrine peptide precursor), whose overexpression reduces POMC levels implicated in appetite and energy expenditure (Del Signore et al., 2004). The effects on mRNA levels may be mediated by glucocorticoid receptors responsible for the negative feedback response (Herman et al., 1989) or indirect vestibular afferents to the hippocampus (Stackman et al., 2002).

In the hippocampus, mice exposed to a 4G load were more susceptible to long-term potentiation (LTP), an electrophysiological index of plasticity or learning, without being affected for basal neurotransmission measured by input-output coupling of Schaffer collaterals (Ishii et al., 2004). This facilitation may be caused by increased phosphorylation of the GluR1 subunit of the amino-hydroxy-methyl-propionic acid (AMPA) receptor observed in these 4G-exposed mice. However, no effect on LTP was discovered in rats exposed to a 2G load for 2 or 14 days (Guinan et al., 1998). Rats exposed to 10G for 5 min inside a centrifuge had higher than normal Terminal deoxynucleotidyl transferase dUTP nick end labeling (TUNEL) staining and caspase-3 activity in the CA1 subregion of the hippocampus as well as impaired spatial learning in the Morris water maze (Feng et al., 2010). The effects of a 7-day exposure to a 2G load on 5HT modulation were measured on hippocampal pathways by recording dentate gyrus and CA1 pyramidal cell layer activity (Horrigan et al., 1997). 5HT decreased the amplitude of the population spike in both subregions of rats exposed to 2G. The 5-HT1A agonist 8-OH-DPAT mimicked this inhibition in both regions of controls. However, 8-OH-DPAT responses were not affected by exposure to 2G.

4. Combined Hypo- and Hypergravity

4.1. Parabolic Flights

To test the hypothesis that altered gravity causes plastic changes in the vestibulo-cardiovascular reflex, arterial pressure and hypothalamic glutamate concentrations were examined in rats maintained under a 3G load or normal gravity for 2 weeks (Morita et al., 2007). The vestibulo-cardiovascular reflex was stimulated by a gravitational change induced by a parabolic flight consisting of 3 phases: "pull-up" during which the G load gradually increased to 2G, a 20s "push-over" into microgravity, and a "pull-out" during which the G load increased. In the 1G group, arterial pressure increased during the pull-up hypergravity period, a response attenuated in the 3G group. During the push-over microgravity period, arterial pressure decreased from peak levels in the pull-up period and recovered to the pre-parabolic level. In the 3G group, arterial pressure was not altered by push-over microgravity. These arterial pressure responses were associated with higher glutamate concentrations in the hypothalamus, also attenuated in the 3G group. Such results indicate that an altered gravitational environment induces plastic alterations in the vestibulo-cardiovascular reflex.

4.2. Simulated Parabolic Flights

The effects of high sustained hypergravity after 7 days of simulated weightlessness were examined on learning and neuronal apoptosis in rats (Sun et al., 2009). Exposure to 15G centrifugation, hindlimb suspension, or both (tail suspension followed by centrifugation) delayed acquisition of light-dark discrimination and passive avoidance tasks. TUNEL staining revealed apoptotic cells in hippocampus and neocortex in hypergravity, simulated weightlessness, and combined groups, and TUNEL positive cells were maximal in the combined group. Furthermore, rats with combined treatment revealed a synergistic effect in Y-maze and passive avoidance tests. These findings indicate that simulated weightlessness may exacerbate hypergravity-induced impairment of learning and memory, perhaps caused by neuronal cell death in the hippocampus.

References

Akima, H; Kawakami, Y; Kubo, K; Sekiguchi, C; Ohshima, H; Miyamoto, A; Fukunaga, T. Effect of short-duration spaceflight on thigh and leg muscle volume. *Med Sci Sports Exerc*, 2000, 32, 1743-7.

Antoni, FA. Hypothalamic control of adrenocorticotropin secretion: advances since the discovery of 41-residue corticotropin-releasing factor. *Endocr Rev*, 1986, 7, 351-78.

Armstrong, WE. Hypothalamic supraopotic and paraventricular nuclei. In: G Paxinos (ed) *The rat nervous system.* Amsterdam: Elsevier, 369-88, 2004.

Besnard, S; Machado, ML; Vignaux, G; Boulouard, M; Coquerel, A; Bouet, V; Freret, T; Denise, P; Lelong-Boulouard, V. Influence of vestibular input on spatial and nonspatial memory and on hippocampal NMDA receptors. *Hippocampus,* 2012, 22, 814-26.

Bodnoff, SR; Humphreys, AG; Lehman, JC; Diamond, DM; Rose, GM; Meaney, MJ. Enduring effects of chronic corticosterone treatment on spatial learning, synaptic plasticity, and hippocampal neuropathology in young and mid-aged rats. *J Neurosci,* 1995, 15, 61-9.

Bruce, LL. Adaptations of the vestibular system to short and long-term exposures to altered gravity. *Adv Space Res,* 2003, 32, 1533-9.

Centini, C; Pompeiano, O. Sleep research in space: expression of immediate early genes in forebrain structures of rats during the NASA neurolab mission (STS-90). *Arch Ital Biol,* 2007, 145, 117-50.

Culman, J; Kvetnansky, T; Serova, LV; Tigranjan, RA; Macho, L. Serotonin in individual hypothalamic nuclei of rats after space flight on biosatellite Cosmos 1129. *Acta Astronaut,* 1985, 12, 373-6.

D'Amelio, F; Wu, LC; Fox, RA; Daunton, NG; Corcoran, ML; Polyakov, I. Hypergravity exposure decreases gamma-aminobutyric acid immunoreactivity in axon terminals contacting pyramidal cells in the rat somatosensory cortex: a quantitative immunocytochemical image analysis. *J Neurosci Res,* 1998, 53, 135-42.

Da Silva, MS; Zimmerman, PM; Meguid, MM; Nandi, J; Ohinata, K; Xu, Y; Chen, C; Tada, T; Inui, A. Anorexia in space and possible etiologies: an overview. *Nutrition,* 2002, 18, 805-13.

Day, JR; Frank, AT; O'Callaghan, JP; DeHart, BW. Effects of microgravity and bone morphogenetic protein II on GFAP in rat brain. *J Appl Physiol,* 1998, 85, 716-22.

Del Signore, A; Mandillo, S; Rizzo, A; Di Mauro, E; Mele, A; Negri, R; Oliverio, A; Paggi, P. Hippocampal gene expression is modulated by hypergravity. *Eur J Neurosci,* 2004, 19, 667-77.

de Quervain, DJ; Roozendaal, B; McGaugh, JL. Stress and glucocorticoids impair retrieval of long-term spatial memory. *Nature,* 1998, 394, 787-90.

Douglas, RJ; Clark, GM; Erway, LC; Hubbard, DG; Wright, CG. Effects of genetic vestibular defects on behavior related to spatial orientation and emotionality. *J Comp Physiol Psychol,* 1979, 93, 467-80.

Fareh, J; Fagette, S; Cottet-Emard, JM; Allevard, AM; Viso, M; Gauquelin, G; Gharib, C. Comparison of the effects of spaceflight and hindlimb-suspension on rat pituitary vasopressin and brainstem norepinephrine content. *Adv Space Res*, 1994, 14, 365-71.

Fareh, J; Cottet-Emard, JM; Pequignot, JM; Jahns, G; Meylor, J; Viso, M; Vassaux, D; Gauquelin, G; Gharib, C. Norepinephrine content in discrete brain areas and neurohypophysial vasopressin in rats after a 9-d spaceflight (SLS-1). *Aviat Space Environ Med*, 1993, 64, 507-11.

Feng, S; Wang, Q; Wang, H; Peng, Y; Wang, L; Lu, Y; Shi, T; Xiong, L. Electroacupuncture pretreatment ameliorates hypergravity-induced impairment of learning and memory and apoptosis of hippocampal neurons in rats. *Neurosci Lett*, 2010, 478, 150-5.

Francia, N; Santucci, D; Chiarotti, F; Alleva, E. Cognitive and emotional alterations in periadolescent mice exposed to 2 g hypergravity field. *Physiol Behav*, 2004, 83, 383-94.

Frigeri, A; Iacobas, DA; Iacobas, S; Nicchia, GP; Desaphy, JF; Camerino, DC; Svelto, M; Spray, DC. Effect of microgravity on gene expression in mouse brain. *Exp Brain Res*, 2008, 191, 289-300.

Fuller, PM; Jones, TA; Jones, SM; Fuller, CA. Evidence for macular gravity receptor modulation of hypothalamic, limbic and autonomic nuclei. *Neuroscience*, 2004, 129, 461-71.

Gauer, OH; Henry, JP; Behn, C. The regulation of extracellular fluid volume. *Annu Rev Physiol*, 1970, 32, 547-95.

Gazenko, OG; Genin, AM; Il'in, EA; Serova, LV; Tigranyan, RA; Oganov, VS. Physiological mechanisms of adaptation to weightlessness. Data from experiments with animals in earth-orbit biosatellites. *Biol Bull Acad Sci USSR*, 1980, 7, 1-12.

Ghelarducci, B. Responses of the cerebellar fastigial neurones to tilt. *Pflugers Arch*, 1973, 344, 195-206.

Goldberg, JM; Wilson, VJ; Cullen, KE. The vestibular system: a sixth sense, chapter 6: Neuroanatomy of central vestibular pathways, 137-190. OxFord: Oxford University Press. 2012.

Guinan, MJ; Horowitz, JM; Fuller, CA. Effects of hyperdynamic fields on input-output relationships and long-term potentiation in the rat hippocampus. *J Gravit Physiol*, 1998, 5, 31-40.

Gustave Dit Duflo, S; Gestreau, C; Lacour, M. Fos expression in the rat brain after exposure to gravito-inertial force changes. *Brain Res*, 2000, 861, 333-44.

Heath, RG; Dempesy, CW; Fontana, CJ; Myers. WA. Cerebellar stimulation: effects on septal region, hippocampus, and amygdala of cats and rats. *Biol Psychiatry*, 1978, 13, 501-29.

Herdegen, T; Leah, JD. Inducible and constitutive transcription factors in the mammalian nervous system: control of gene expression by Jun, Fos and Krox, and CREB/ATF proteins. *Brain Res Rev*, 1998, 28, 370-490.

Herman, JP; Schäfer, MK; Young, EA; Thompson, R; Douglass, J; Akil, H; Watson, SJ. Evidence for hippocampal regulation of neuroendocrine neurons of the hypothalamo-pituitary-adrenocortical axis. *J Neurosci*, 1989, 9, 3072-82.

Horii, A; Nakagawa, A; Uno, A; Kitahara, T; Imai, T; Nishiike, S; Takeda, N; Inohara, H. Implication of substance P neuronal system in the amygdala as a possible mechanism for hypergravity-induced motion sickness. *Brain Res*, 2012, 1435, 91-8.

Horrigan, DJ; Fuller, CA; Horowitz, JM. Effects of hypergravic fields on serotonergic neuromodulation in the rat hippocampus. *J Gravit Physiol*, 1997, 4, 21-30.

Ishii, M; Tomizawa, K; Matsushita, M; Matsui, H. Exposure of mouse to high gravitation forces induces long-term potentiation in the hippocampus. *Acta Med Okayama*, 2004, 58, 143-9.

Katafuchi, T; Koizumi, K. Fastigial inputs to paraventricular neurosecretory neurones studied by extra- and intracellular recordings in rats. *J Physiol*, 1990, 421, 535-51.

Katafuchi, T; Oomura, Y; Aoyagi, K. Single neuron activity of rat hypothalamic paraventricular nucleus during body suspension. *Neurosci Lett*, 1987, 78, 301-6.

Katafuchi, T; Hori, T; Oomura, Y; Koizumi, K. Cerebellar afferents to neuroendocrine cells: implications for adaptive responses to simulated weightlessness. *Endocr J*, 1995, 42, 729-37.

Kirkby, RJ; Stein, DG; Kimble, RJ; Kimble, DP. Effects of hippocampal lesions and duration of sensory input on spontaneous alternation. *J Comp Physiol Psychol*, 1967, 64, 342-5.

Kumei, Y; Toda, K; Kawauchi, Y; Shimokawa, R; Shimokawa, H; Makita, K. Nociceptive responses and immunohistochemical changes in the rat brain under gravity stress. *J Gravit Physiol*, 2000, 7, P91-2.

Kumei, Y; Shimokawa, R; Kimoto, M; Kawauchi, Y; Shimokawa, H; Makita, K; Ohya, K; Toda, K. Gravity stress elevates the nociceptive threshold level with immunohistochemical changes in the rat brain. *Acta Astronaut*, 2001, 49, 381-90.

Kumei, Y; Shimokawa, R; Toda, K; Kawauchi, Y; Makita, K; Terasawa, M; Ohya, K; Shimokawa, H. Hypergravity modulates behavioral nociceptive responses in rats. *Adv Space Res*, 2002, 30, 783-8.

Kvetnansky, R; Culman, J; Serova, LV; Tigranjan, RA; Torda, T; Macho, L. Catecholamines and their enzymes in discrete brain areas of rats after space flight on biosatellites Cosmos. *Acta Astronaut*, 1983, 10, 295-300.

Lalonde, R. The neurobiological basis of spontaneous alternation. *Neurosci Biobeh Rev*, 2002, 26, 91-104.

Lew, PS; Wong, D; Yamaguchi, T; Leckstrom, A; Schwartz, J; Dodd, JG; Mizuno, TM. Tail suspension increases energy expenditure independently of the melanocortin system in mice. *Can J Physiol Pharmacol*, 2009, 87, 839-49.

Machado, ML; Kroichvili, N; Freret, T; Philoxène, B; Lelong-Boulouard, V; Denise, P; Besnard, S. Spatial and non-spatial performance in mutant mice devoid of otoliths. *Neurosci Lett*, 2012, 522, 57-61.

Mandillo, S; Del Signore, A; Paggi, P; Francia, N; Santucci, D; Mele, A; Oliverio, A. Effects of acute and repeated daily exposure to hypergravity on spatial learning in mice. *Neurosci Lett*, 2003, 336, 147-50.

Mitani, K; Horii, A; Kubo, T. Impaired spatial learning after hypergravity exposure in rats. *Cogn Brain Res*, 2004, 22, 94-100.

Morey-Holton, ER; Globus, RK. Hindlimb unloading rodent model: technical aspects. *J Appl Physiol*, 2002, 92, 1367-77.

Morita, H; Abe, C; Awazu, C; Tanaka, K. Long-term hypergravity induces plastic alterations in vestibulo-cardiovascular reflex in conscious rats. *Neurosci Lett*, 2007, 412, 201-5.

Murakami, DM; Tang, IH; Fuller, CA. Chronic 2G exposure affects c-Fos reactivity to a light pulse within the rat suprachiasmatic nucleus. *J Gravit Physiol*, 1998, 5, 71-8.

Nakagawa, A; Uno, A; Horii, A; Kitahara, T; Kawamoto, M; Uno, Y; Fukushima, M; Nishiike, S; Takeda, N; Kubo, T. Fos induction in the amygdala by vestibular information during hypergravity stimulation. *Brain Res*, 2003, 986, 114-23.

Ordy, JM; Brizzee, KR; Samorajski, T. The effects of cosmic particle radiation on pocket mice aboard Apollo XVII: appendix I. Condition of flight animals on recovery; food intake; observations on hypothalamus, pituitary, and adrenal glands. *Aviat Space Environ Med*, 1975, 46, 627-33.

Palkovitz, J. Afferents onto neuroendocrine cells. In: D Ganten, D Pfaff (eds) *Morphology of hypothalamus and its connections*. Berlin: Springer-Verlag, 197-222, 1986.

Perciavalle, V; Berretta, S; Raffaele, R. Projections from the intracerebellar nuclei to the ventral midbrain tegmentum in the rat. *Neuroscience*, 1989, 29, 109-19.

Pompeiano, O. Contribution of REM sleep to Fos and FRA expression in the vestibular nuclei of rat leading to vestibular adaptation during the STS-90 Neurolab Mission. *Arch Ital Biol*, 2007, 145, 55-85.

Pompeiano, O; d'Ascanio, P; Balaban, E; Centini, C; Pompeiano, M. Gene expression in autonomic areas of the medulla and the central nucleus of the amygdala in rats during and after space flight. *Neuroscience*, 2004, 124, 53-69.

Ricardo, JA; Koh, ET. Anatomical evidence of direct projections from the nucleus of the solitary tract to the hypothalamus, amygdala, and other forebrain structures in the rat. *Brain Res*, 1978, 153, 1-26.

Roberts, WW; Dember, WN; Brodwick, M. Alternation and exploration in rats with hippocampal lesions. *J Comp Physiol Psychol*, 1962, 55, 695-700.

Roozendaal, B; Griffith, QK; Buranday, J; De Quervain, DJ; McGaugh, JL. The hippocampus mediates glucocorticoid-induced impairment of spatial memory retrieval: dependence on the basolateral amygdala. *Proc Natl Acad Sci USA*, 2003, 100, 1328-33.

Saper, CB; Loewy, AD. Efferent connections of the parabrachial nucleus in the rat. *Brain Res*, 1980, 197, 291-317.

Sarkar, P; Sarkar, S; Ramesh, V; Kim, H; Barnes, S; Kulkarni, A; Hall, JC; Wilson, BL; Thomas, RL; Pellis, NR; Ramesh, GT. Proteomic analysis of mouse hypothalamus under simulated microgravity. *Neurochem Res*, 2008, 33, 2335-41.

Sato, G; Uno, A; Horii, A; Umehara, H; Kitamura, Y; Sekine, K; Tamura, K; Fukui, H; Takeda, N. Effects of hypergravity on histamine H1 receptor mRNA expression in hypothalamus and brainstem of rats: implications for development of motion sickness. *Acta Otolaryngol*, 2009, 129, 45-51.

Schneider, S; Guardiera, S; Abel, T; Carnahan, H; Strüder, HK. Artificial gravity results in changes in frontal lobe activity measured by EEG tomography. *Brain Res*, 2009, 1285, 119-26.

Simerly, RB. Anatomic substrates of hypothalamic integration In: G Paxinos (ed) *The rat nervous system.* Amsterdam: Elsevier, 335-68, 2004.

Smith, PF; Zheng, Y. From ear to uncertainty: vestibular contributions to cognitive functions. *Front Neurosci*, 2013, 84, 1-13.

Smith, PF; Horii, A; Russell, N; Bilkey, N; Zheng, Y; Liu, P; Kerr, S; Darlington, CL. The effects of vestibular lesions on hippocampal function in rats. *Prog Neurobiol*, 2005, 75, 391-405.

Snider, RS; Maiti, A. Cerebellar contributions to the Papez circuit. *J Neurosci Res*, 1976, 2, 133-46.

Snider, RS; Maiti, A; Snider, SR. Cerebellar pathways to ventral midbrain and nigra. *Exp Neurol*, 1976, 53, 714-28.

Stackman, RW; Clark, AS; Taube, JS. Hippocampal spatial representations require vestibular input. *Hippocampus*, 2002, 12, 291-303.

Stein, TP; Schluter, MD. Excretion of IL-6 by astronauts during spaceflight. *Am J Physiol*, 1994, 266, E448-52.

Sun, XQ; Xu, ZP; Zhang, S; Cao, XS; Liu, TS. Simulated weightlessness aggravates hypergravity-induced impairment of learning and memory and neuronal apoptosis in rats. *Behav Brain Res*, 2009, 199, 197-202.

Tai, SK; Leung, S. Vestibular stimulation enhances hippocampal long-term potentiation via activation of cholinergic septohippocampal cells. *Behav Brain Res*, 2012, 232, 174-82.

Temple, MD; Kosik, KS; Steward, O. Spatial learning and memory is preserved in rats after early development in a microgravity environment. *Neurobiol Learn Mem*, 2002, 78, 199-216.

Tracy, AL; Jarrard, LE; Davidson, TL. The hippocampus and motivation revisited: appetite and activity. *Behav Brain Res*, 2001, 127, 13-23.

Uno, A; Takeda, N; Horii, A; Morita, M; Yamamoto, Y; Yamatodani, A; Kubo, T. Histamine release from the hypothalamus induced by gravity change in rats and space motion sickness. *Physiol Behav*, 1997, 61, 883-7.

Uno, A; Takeda, N; Horii, A; Sakata, Y; Yamatodani, A; Kubo, T. Effects of amygdala or hippocampus lesion on hypergravity-induced motion sickness in rats. *Acta Otolaryngol.*, 2000, 120, 860-5.

Vidal, P-P; Sans, A. Vestibular system. In: G Paxinos (ed) *The rat nervous system.* Amsterdam: Elsevier, 965-96, 2004.

Wise, KC; Manna, SK; Yamauchi, K; Ramesh, V; Wilson, BL; Thomas, RL; Sarkar, S; Kulkarni, AD; Pellis, NR; Ramesh, GT. Activation of nuclear transcription factor-kappaB in mouse brain induced by a simulated microgravity environment. *In Vitro Cell Dev Biol Anim*, 2005, 41, 118-23.

Chapter 4

Limbic System Alterations in Opioid Addiction

Anna G. Polunina**[*] **and Evgeny A. Bryun
Moscow Research and Practical Center for Narcology,
Department of Healthcare of Moscow, Russia

Abstract

Anterior cingulate cortex, amygdala and insular cortex are characterized by very high concentration of mu-opioid receptors, and enkephalin is the most abundant opioid agonist in these limbic system structures. Neuroimaging studies of healthy subjects consistently showed activation of limbic cortex and subcortical structures after mu-opioid agonist injection, and involvement of opioid innervation of limbic structures into generation of positive emotions, control of pain and negative emotions. Experimental and clinical studies demonstrated that chronic administration of pharmacological opioid agonists induced profound remodeling of brain structures supporting reward and emotion processing. Chronic opioid treatment strengthened interneuronal connections involved into opioid-seeking behaviors, whereas processing of non-drug-related rewards and emotions is deficient in addicted animals and humans.

[*] Corresponding author: Dr. Anna Polunina, 101 − 8 − 7 Pr-t Vernadskogo Moscow 119526 Russia. Tel./Fax: +7-916-129-19-80, E-mail: anpolunina@mail.ru.

Besides neuroplastic changes in limbic structures, opioid receptor signaling and endogenous opioid ligands production are impaired after chronic opioid treatment. In contrast to animal studies, clinical studies of opioid addiction register not only the neuropsychiatric effects of the drug, but also premorbid abnormalities. A range of studies demonstrated high prevalence of conduct disorder, antisocial personality disorder and depression in opioid addicts, and all these neuropsychiatric conditions are characterized by dysfunctional limbic neuronetworks. Although, neuropsychiatric traits are premorbid in many opioid addicts, chronic drug abuse worsens the neuropsychiatric status within the course of the addiction or induces newly developed psychiatric abnormalities.

Keywords: Amygdala, anterior cingulate cortex, emotion, heroin

Introduction

Chronic opioid abuse induces progressive neuropsychiatric phenomena, which include acute opioid withdrawal syndrome, craving and protracted opioid abstinence symptoms, and inevitable personality changes.

Recent studies showed that prominent emotional and autonomic innervation disturbances in opioid addicts relate to dysfunction of limbic cortical and subcortical structures.

The present review is focused on anterior cingulate cortex (ACC) and amygdale dysfunction in opioid addicts as these structures of limbic system are most densely innervated by mu-opioid receptors, and their functions have been studied most intensively. Opioid innervation of ACC and amygdala is involved into neurocircuits processing emotion, autonomic control, and nociception, and to a lesser degree attention and memory. The experimental and clinical studies of the neuropsychiatric abnormalities in opioid addiction are summarized in the present review as well.

Opioid Innervation of Limbic Structures

Opioid Innervation of Limbic Structures

In humans, amygdala, ACC and insular cortex, are characterized by very high concentration of opioid receptors, which is similar to basal ganglia and is only a little bit lower in comparison with thalamus (Baumgärtner et al., 2006;

Vogt et al., 2004). In other mammals, mu-opioid receptors are densely distributed in ACC (especially perigenual cortex) and amygdale as well (Le Merrer et al., 2009; Mansour et al., 1988; Vogt et al., 2001). The distribution of delta -receptors is most abundant in layers 1 and 2 of the neocortex and amygdala (Penney, 1996). In contrast to mu- receptors, delta-opioid receptors bind densely in the hippocampal formation, particularly in the dentate gyrus. Overall, delta- opioid receptors predominate in forebrain structures, such as neocortex and amygdala (Mansour et al., 1988).

Within human cingulate cortex the highest binding of opioid receptors was reported in the posterior region of anterior cingulate cortex with lesser amounts in middle cingulate cortex, and the least in posterior cingulate cortex (Vogt et al., 2004).

Opioid receptors in cingulate cortex regulate predominantly motor and motivation behaviors, including nociception during motor activity, and many of the cortical motor projection systems arise in layer V where there are the highest level of opioid receptor binding and the most nociceptive neurons. The sources of opioid receptors in the cingulate cortex include locus coeruleus and thalamic nuclei, where from considerable proportion of opioid receptors is transported to cingulate cortex (Vogt et al., 2004).

Enkephalin is the most abundant opioid agonist in anterior cingulate cortex, insular cortex and amygdale (Mansour et al., 1988; Penney, 1996; Vogt et al., 2001; Evans et al., 2007). Although encephalin has ten-fold higher affinities for delta-receptors than for mu-receptors, its ability to activate mu-receptors is considerable and dose-related (Penney, 1996; Vogt et al., 2001). Overall, met-enkephalinergic neurons are suggested to be the primary source of peptide that activates mu-opioid receptors in anterior cingulate cortex, and met-enkephalinergic neurons are found throughout ACC (Vogt et al., 2001).

It should be noted, that opioids and other neuropeptides are more slowly degraded and are therefore able to diffuse much greater distances in comparison with classical neurotransmitters (Knoll et al., 2010). This mode of action enables neuropeptides to convey information and coordinate activity across broader networks of neurons.

Neuroimaging studies of healthy subjects consistently showed activation of limbic cortex and subcortical structures after mu-opioid agonist injection, whereas sensory and dorsolateral prefrontal cortex tended to deactivate in this condition (Becerra et al., 2006; Leppä et al., 2006; Mac Intosh et al., 2008; Khalili-Mahani et al., 2011). The activation of anterior cingulate cortex after mu- agonists was shown both in healthy subjects (Leppä et al., 2006; Mac Intosh et al., 2008; Khalili-Mahani et al., 2011) and opioid addicts (Schlaepfer et al., 1998). In the study of Khalili-Mahani et al. (2011) the pregenual ACC was one of the regions which showed the highest increase in absolute cerebral blood flow after morphine injection.

Nevertheless, Becerra and colleagues (2006) reported deactivation of anterior cingulate cortex after low doses of morphine.

Other brain structures, which were shown to be activated by systemic opioid agonists included insular cortex, operculum, amygdale, orbitofrontal cortex, hippocampus, nucleus accumbens, putamen, hypothalamus, and substantia nigra (Becerra et al., 2006; Leppä et al., 2006; Mac Intosh et al., 2008; Khalili-Mahani et al., 2011).

Functional Role of Opioid Innervation of Limbic Structures

Neuroimaging studies of normal subjects consistently demonstrated involvement of opioid innervation of limbic structures into generating of positive emotion, control of pain and negative emotions.

The role of opioid innervations in autonomic regulation and attention/ memory functions is less clear.

Petrovic and colleagues (2008) studied effects of naloxone administration to healthy subjects before Gambling test. Under the influence of naloxone, subjects rated rewards as less pleasurable. In the loss condition, subjects rated negative outcomes as more aversive after naloxone compared to placebo, and this negative trend were related to enhanced activity in caudal ACC and anterior insula after naloxone. In placebo condition, both larger rewards and larger losses were associated with enhanced activity in rostral region of ACC, however, naloxone attenuated these effects of reinforcement magnitude both for losses and rewards. The authors concluded that the outcome magnitude-related activation in rostral ACC may be associated with opioid regulation of the hedonic experience in rewards and countering the aversive experience of losses.

In normal subjects, the sustained sadness condition (focusing on an autobiographical event associated with a profound feeling of sadness) was consistently shown to be associated with deactivation of mu-opioid neurotransmission in limbic structures, including rostral ACC and amygdala (Prossin et al., 2010; Kennedy et al., 2006; Zubieta et al., 2003). In contrast to healthy controls, patients with major depression and borderline personality disorder tended to demonstrate activation of opioid innervation in pregenual

ACC, amygdale and other structures during sadness condition (Prossin et al., 2010; Kennedy et al., 2006).

Involvement of ACC into pain control is well established, and this function is realized by tight interaction of limbic and motor structures (Zubieta and Stohler, 2009).

For instance, motor cortex stimulation is a valuable approach for pain relief, and recently it was shown that chronic motor cortex stimulation induces significant changes in opioid innervation of anterior middle cingulate cortex and periaqueductal gray, correlating with pain relief (Maarrawi et al., 2007). In addition, Mueller et al. (2010) showed lower opioid receptors availability in left inferior frontal, anterior cingulate and insular cortex and higher cold pain-sensitivity in normal subjects.

The same study showed significant association between lower opioid receptor availability in motor and premotor areas and stronger perception of cold-related pain. High pain rating index was associated with opioid binding decrease in midcingulate and ipsilateral temporal cortex in patients with chronic neuropathic pain in the study of Klega and colleagues (2010).

The investigations of the role of rich opioid innervation of amygdale have only recently been started. Mahler and Berridge (2009) showed that activation of mu- opioid neurotransmission in central nuclei of amygdale enhanced appetitive and consummatory behaviors directed toward each animal's own prepotent conditional stimulus.

Overall, the abundant amygdalar opioid innervation is considered as a cue region of stress response and anxiety level regulation by many researchers (Randall-Thompson et al., 2010; Chieng et al., 2006; Beckerman and Glass, 2012). Chieng and colleagues (2006) showed that the mu-opioid receptor agonist (DAMGO) induced inhibition of 61% of cells in the central amygdala. The researchers concluded that opioids can directly inhibit output from the amygdale by activating distinct subpopulations of opioid-sensitive neurons.

Precise functional role of delta-opioid innervation of hippocampus remains unclear (Penney et al., 1996; Le Merrer et al., 2009). In animals it was shown that application of morphine or beta-endorphin disrupted interneuron network gamma oscillations in hippocampus.

Whittington and colleagues (1998) concluded that opioid agonists may disturb cognition via disruption of interneuron network oscillations.

At the same time, Rodefer and Nguyen (2008) reported improvement of attention-set shifting in aged rats after naltrexone administration with no effect of naltrexone in young rats.

Moreover, at least three studies showed enhancing effects of mu-/delta-opioid innervation on memory via modulation of attention-related responses and learning (Chaves et al., 1988; Hernandez et al., 1997; Holahan et al., 2008). Chaves and colleagues (1988) observed enhancing effect of novel experiences on performance in memory tests in untreated and placebo-treated healthy subjects. At the same time, administration of naltrexone blocked the enhancing effect of novel experience on memory, and this finding evidence that endogenous opioids are involved in cognitive processing.

Hence, mu- opioid innervation is dense in anterior and middle cingulate cortex and amygdale, and enkephalin is the main endogenous opioid agonist at this region.

The main functions of opioid innervation of cingulate cortex include positive emotion generation and control of pain and negative emotions.

Opioid innervation of amygdale is involved into inhibition of anxiety and therefore facilitating appetitive and consummatory behaviors. The functional role of delta-opioid innervations of hippocampus remains unclear, and data concerning involvement of endogenous opioids into cognitive activities are controversial.

Limbic System Alterations in Opioid Addiction

Experimental and clinical studies consistently showed that chronic administration of pharmacological opioid agonists induce profound remodeling of brain structures supporting reward and emotion processing.

These alterations are not toxic or neurodegenerative, but neuroplastic, and perhaps at least partially reversible.

Nevertheless, chronic opioids induced alterations in brain connectivity have an evitable and dramatic impact on behaviors of an addicted individual with almost complete reorganization of life priorities and values in comparison with the pre-addictive period.

Experimental Studies

Chronic administration of pharmacological opioids induces profound neuroplastic changes in brain regions involved into reward processing and limbic system structures (Morozov and Bogolepov, 1984; Robinson et al., 2004; Ballesteros-Yáñez et al., 2007).

Morozov and Bogolepov (1984) observed prominent reorganization of cortex dendritic spines with formation of multiple new synapses and destruction of older ones during the first month of daily morphine administration to laboratory rats. Importantly, after the first month of chronic morphine destructive processes prevailed and density of cortex dendritic spines decreased in that study.

These data are in agreement with the findings of Robinson et al. (2002).

The authors reported decrease of dendritic spines density in nucleus accumbens shell, medial frontal (Cg3) and occipital cortex, and oppositely increase of dendritic branching in orbito-frontal cortex in animals after several weeks of morphine treatment. Self-administration and passive administration of the opiate agonist induced somewhat regionally different brain changes along with more prominent dendritic density increase in orbital cortex in self-administering animals in comparison with passive-administering ones. The study of Ballesteros-Yanez et al. (2007) showed enlargement of basal dendritic arbors of medial frontal (Cg3) pyramidal neurons along with reduction in the size and branching complexity of the dendritic arbors of pyramidal cells in the motor cortex in rats chronically treated by morphine.

Overall, the cited studies showed profound neuroplastic reorganization of neural networks in reward processing and limbic structures in animals after chronic exposure to morphine.

Anterior cingulate cortex and amygdale are important components of extensive cortical-subcortical network supporting appetitive learning mechanisms (Pavlovian conditioning) (Everitt et al., 2001; Koob and Volkow, 2010).

Within this network anterior cingulate cortex and amygdale are anatomically and functionally interconnected with the nucleus accumbens and the mesolimbic dopaminergic system.

Neuroplastic changes in appetitive behavior neuronetwork are widely recognized as the core neurological substrate of addiction behaviors (Everitt et al., 2001; Koob and Volkow, 2010). For instance, Li and colleagues (2008) reported increased metabolic processes in central amygdala nucleus in rats after chronic morphine treatment which correlated with increased drug-seeking behaviors.

Inhibition of metabolic processes in central amygdala nucleus decreased drug-seeking, and stimulation of excitatory NMDA neurotransmission in central amygdale induced increase of drug-seeking in the same study. At the same time, Hellemans and colleages (2006) showed involvement of basolateral amygdale into the conditioned heroin withdrawal memories consolidation.

Being involved into processing of drug-related behaviors, limbic structures in addicted animals were shown to be deficient for supporting normal learning processes. Haris and Aston-Jones (2003) showed that during protracted abstinence (2 – 5 weeks) morphine-depended rats were slower during learning about environmental cues that predicted food reinforcement, while at the same time the animals learned normally about cues predictive of morphine reward. The deficit of learning about food reinforcement was not related to a lack of desire for food as the morphine-dependent animals consumed all of the food they were given.

It should be noted, that inhibitory effects of chronic morphine on neurogenesis in dentate gyrus of hippocampus were shown as well. In the study of Eisch et al. (2000), rats receiving morphine for 4 weeks showed 47% fewer newly born cells in the granule layer of the dentate gyrus in comparison with controls. Moreover, Sklair-Tavron et al. (1996) demonstrated that chronic morphine treatment induced 25% reduction of the area and perimeter of dopamine neurons in ventral tegmental area (VTA), which are tightly involved into the mediation of reward learning (Schultz, 1999). Interestingly, that concomitant treatment of rats with either naltrexone or brain-derived neurotrophic factor prevented the reduction of the dopamine neurons in the same study. The authors suggested that structural alterations in VTA neurons could reflect an impairment in the functional capacity of these cells.

The data concerning the opioid receptor function in opioid addiction are controversial. The majority of studies in this field showed functional uncoupling of mu-receptors from cellular signaling pathways rather than global decrease of mu- or delta-opioid receptor density in opioid-dependent animals (Williams et al., 2001; Le Merrer et al., 2009). In the study of Sim-Selley and colleagues (2000), prominent desensitization of mu-receptor-activated G-proteins in morphine-treated animals was registered in brain structures mediating analgesia, autonomic regulation and emotional responses (periaqueductal gray, thalamus, parabrachial nucleus, commissural nucleus tractus solitaries, locus coeruleus, amygdale), whereas effects of chronic heroin in forebrain structures (caudate putamen, cingulated cortex and nucleus accumbens) were small or negligible in the same study. At the same time most studies reported downregulation of proenkephlin mRNA in striatum and other brain regions (hypothalamus, frontal cortex, brainstem nuclei) after chronic morphine treatment (Le Merrer et al., 2009).

Hence, the cited animal studies consistently showed that opioid addiction is characterized by considerable neuroplastic remodeling of limbic structures. Chronic opioids strengthen interneuronal connections involved into opioid-seeking behaviors, whereas processing of non-drug-related rewards is deficient in addicted animals. Besides neuroplastic changes in reward processing and limbic structures, opioid receptor signaling and endogenous opioid ligands production are impaired after chronic opioid treatment.

Human Studies

Childhood Neuropsychiatric Abnormalities in Opioid Addicts

In contrast to animal studies, clinical studies of opioid addiction register not only the neurological effects of the drug, but also premorbid neurological abnormalities.

Retrospective studies consistently found increased frequency of childhood attention-deficit hyperactivity disorder (ADHD) symptoms in opioid addicts prior to drug abuse career (Modestin et al., 2001; Davids et al., 2005). In the study of Davids and colleagues (2005) 29% of opioid-dependent patients reached cut-off points of childhood ADHD syndrome.

This subgroup of patients was characterized by increased rate of dropout of school and higher number of documented antisocial and criminal behaviors in comparison with controls.

Modestin and colleagues (2001) studied frequency of both childhood ADHD and CD in opioid-dependent patients. ADHD alone was found in 4% of patients, ADHD+CD in 7% of patients, CD alone was the most frequent disorder and was registered in 47% of patients. Patients with childhood ADHD were characterized by younger age of the first drug use and less frequent professional qualification in comparison with patients without ADHD. It's logical, that patients with CD were characterized by more frequent violation of laws. At the same time, opioid addicts without CD reported current depression and history of alcohol abuse significantly more frequently in comparison with CD patients. About 20-30% of opioid addicts were reported to reach criteria of antisocial personality disorder as only about a half of subjects with CD in childhood develop antisocial personality disorder (Modestin et al., 2001; Gerra et al., 2014).

Multiple studies showed diminished global grey and white matter volume in children and adult subjects with ADHD (Castellanos et al., 2002; Seidman et al., 2005), and deficits of grey matter in limbic structures (e.g. amygdale, insular and orbitofrontal cortex, etc.) in subjects with conduct disorder and antisocial personality disorder (de Oliveira-Souza et al., 2008; Fairchild et al., 2011; Sterzer et al., 2007).

Functional neuroimaging studies showed insufficient activation of amygdale, insular, orbital and anterior cingulate cortex during emotional information processing in subjects with conduct disorder and antisocial personality disorder as well (Finger et al., 2011; Passamonti et al., 2010; Sterzer et al., 2005).

In addition, sympathetic innervation deficits with decreased heart rate and skin conductance were reported in subjects with conduct disorder or antisocial personality disorder (Frick and Morris, 2004; Ortiz and Raine, 2004; Raine et al., 2000).

Insufficient response of sympathetic innervation to negative emotional stimuli were characteristic for psychopathic subjects as well (Decety et al., 2009; Richell et al., 2003). Hence, the contemporary studies have consistently shown that many opioid addicts are characterized by premorbid limbic system dysfunction.

Current Neuropsychiatric Abnormalities in Opioid Addicts

The majority of drug abusers demonstrate abnormal attitudes, relation-ships and behavior besides using illicit drugs.

Typical behavior problems in opioid addiction include proneness to stealing and forging documents, driving under the influence of any substance, unprotected sexual behavior and trading sex for drugs, academic under-achievement (Subrama-niam et al., 2009). Psychological assessments typically register increased novelty seeking and decreased self-directedness scores in opioid addicts in comparison with controls (Cohen et al., 2005).

In the study of Subramaniam and colleagues (2009) 83% of opioid addicts reached criteria of any DSM-IV psychiatric disorder besides opioid addiction. Cohen and colleagues (2005) observed higher scores on nine scales of Millon Clinical Multi-Axial Inventory in heroin-dependent subjects receiving metha-done maintenance therapy in comparison with healthy controls, and on 13 scales in heroin-dependent subjects withdrawn from methadone maintenance therapy in comparison with controls.

Depression and anxiety are commonly elevated in drug abusers, including opioid addict populations (Bauer et al., 2001; Suh et al., 2009; Gerra et al., 2014).

In the study of Bauer et al. (2001) the mean Beck depression inventory (BDI) score was 11.2 ± 7.4 and Spielberger state anxiety score was 40.6 ± 9.9

in opioid addicts. Major depression episodes were reported by 40% of opioid addicts in the study of Subramaniam et al. (2009), and by 23% of patients in the study of Gerra et al. (2014).

Generalized anxiety symptoms were found in 20% of opioid addicts, and mean score of anxiety was significantly increased in heroin addicts in comparison with controls in the study of Gerra et al. (2014).

Although, neuropsychiatric traits are premorbid in many opioid addicts, chronic drug abuse worsens the neuropsychiatric status within the course of the addiction or induces newly developed psychiatric abnormalities.

For instance, in the study of Stevens and colleagues (2001) 25.6% of 121 substance abusers reached criteria of antisocial personality disorder, but did not demonstrate conduct disorder during childhood. The authors suggested that antisocial behaviors were a consequence of regular drug abuse in the former patient cohort, and that adolescent brain may be more vulnerable to the effects of addictive substances because of the extensive neuromaturational processes that are occurring during this period.

Importantly, the presence of neuropsychiatric abnormalities may be an important predictor of treatment outcome (Cohen et al., 2005).

In the study of Cohen and colleagues (2005) patients withdrawn from methadone maintenance therapy demonstrated elevated scores on the schizoid, paranoid, aggressive-sadistic, dependent and delusional disorder scales in comparison with patients which were stabilized at methadone maintenance. In our study, individual variability of cognitive performance was significantly associated with the amount of heroin, which patients self-administered per day before admission to the in-patient unit (Bryun et al., 2002).

Hence, both premorbid and newly developed neupsychiatric abnormalities may contribute to unfavorable course of opioid abuse and treatment outcomes.

Neuroimaging Studies

Limbic system and reward processing structures function abnormally in opioid addicts during resting state. Galynker et al. (2000) observed significantly higher glucose metabolism in bilateral anterior cingulate hyrus in methadone maintained and methadone withdrawn opiate-dependent subjects in comparison with controls. Ma and colleagues (2010) showed significantly stronger functional connectivity between ventral/rostral ACC and nucleus accumbens (NAc), between amygdale and lateral orbitofronal cortex (OFC), between NAc and medial OFC, between lateral OFC and medial OFC, and within medial OFC in heroin addicts in comparison with controls.

At the same time significantly weaker functional connectivity was found between dorsal ACC and ventral/rostral ACC, between dorsal ACC and dorsolateral PFC, within lateral OFC, between OFC and some frontal and parietal regions.

Not surprisingly, abnormally increased mu-opioid receptor binding potential in ACC, ventral caudate/NAc and inferior prefrontal cortex was demonstrated in opioid addicts as well (Zubieta et al., 2000).

During induction of craving by the heroin-related cue-exposure opiate-dependent subjects demonstrate significant activation of limbic structures (Daglish et al., 2001, 2003; Zijlstra et al., 2009). Daglish et al. (2001, 2003) observed significant increase of regional cerebral blood flow in the left medial prefrontal region and adjacent left anterior cingulate cortex during drug-related stimulus. In addition, crave/urge scale score significantly correlated with the activation in left orbitofrontal cortex in the same study.

Interestingly, activity in ACC was significantly associated with activity in the left temporal region during craving, whereas the left OFC region activity correlated with activity in the right OFC, left parietal and posterior insular regions, hippocampus and brainstem.

Similar findings were reported in the study of Zijlstra and colleagues (2009), which showed activation of amygdale, bilateral hippocampal region and subcortical nuclei (putamen, right thalamus and right subthalamic nucleus) during viewing heroin-related stimuli in recently detoxified opiate-dependent subjects in contrast to controls. Activation of bilateral amygdale, right subthalamic nucleus and ventral tegmentum area was significantly associated with the severity of the acute heroin craving in opioid-dependent subjects.

Being hyperresponsive to opiate-related cues, limbic structures in opioid addicts are deficient in processing non-drug related emotional and cognitive information.

In the study of Zijstra and colleagues (2009), opioid addicts did not demonstrate activation of limbic structures (bilateral posterior hippocampus, dorsal anterior cingulate cortex, right insula), bilateral dorsomedial prefrontal cortex and subcortical nuclei (putamen, left globus pallidus, caudate nucleus, subthalamic nucleus) during viewing pleasant stimuli in contrast to controls, whereas anhedonia scores inversely correlated with activation of ACC and prefrontal cortex in both groups. Wang et al. (2010) reported reduced activation in right amygdale in response to the affective pictures in opioid addicts in comparison with controls. Martin-Soelch and colleagues (2001) found activation of meso-striatal and meso-corticolimbic sircuits in opioid addicts only in response to monetary reward in contrast to controls, which responded by activations of these neurocircuites to both monetary and non-monetary rewards. Forman et al. (2004) observed attenuated anterior cingulate cortex error signal during memory task and significantly poorer task performance in opiate addicts in comparison with controls.

Overall, the authors of the cited studies concluded that drug-related stimuli activate neurocircuites to a greater degree than non-drug related stimuli in opiate addicts.

Depression and anxiety related neuroimaging abnormalities in opioid addicts were reported as well. Suh and colleagues (2009) found significantly decreased activity of bilateral ventrolateral prefrontal cortex and middle frontal gyri, and left inferior parietal cortex in opioid addicts with moderately increased BDI scores.

These data are consistent with previous studies of non-drug abusing depressive patients. In the study of Wang and colleagues (2010) opioid addicts showed greater activation of visual cortex in response to negative versus positive affective stimuli, whereas controls showed the opposite pattern.

Abnormal functioning of sympathetic innervation and hypothalamus-pituitary-adrenal axis was demonstrated in opioid addicts (Kapoor et al., 1993; Gerra et al., 2004, 2014). Kapoor and colleagues (1993) reported increased heart rate and galvanic skin resistance, and decreased blood pressure in addicts currently using heroin (in 2 − 6 hours after injection of low dose of the drug). In the study of Gerra et al. (2004) abstinent heroin addicts (length of complete abstinence more than 6 months) were characterized by normal heart rate, blood pressure, norepinephrine and epinephrine levels at baseline.

At the same time, basal levels of cortisol and adrenocorticotropic hormone (ACTH) were significantly higher in heroin-dependent patients in comparison with controls in the same study. In addition, the response of sympathetic innervation during negative emotional condition was significantly higher in heroin addicts in comparison with the controls (significantly higher increase of heart rate, systolic blood pressure, and norepinephrine and epinephrine levels).

In contrast to catecholamines, heroin addicts showed significantly smaller increase of cortisol and ACTH with significantly smaller levels of the hormones during negative emotional loading in comparison with the controls.

Conclusion

Anterior cingulate cortex, amygdala and insular cortex are characterized by very high concentration of mu-opioid receptors, and enkephalin is the most abundant opioid agonist in these limbic system structures. Neuroimaging studies of healthy subjects consistently showed activation of limbic cortex and subcortical structures after mu-opioid agonist injection, and involvement of opioid innervation of limbic structures into generation of positive emotions, control of pain and negative emotions. Experimental and clinical studies demonstrated that chronic administration of pharmacological opioid agonists induced profound remodeling of brain structures supporting reward and emotion processing. Chronic opioid treatment strengthened interneuronal connections involved into opioid-seeking behaviors, whereas processing of non-drug-related rewards and emotions is deficient in addicted animals and humans. Besides neuroplastic changes in reward processing and limbic structures, opioid receptor signaling and endogenous opioid ligands production are impaired after chronic opioid treatment. In contrast to animal studies, clinical studies of opioid addiction register not only the neuropsychiatric effects of the drug, but also premorbid abnormalities.

A range of studies demonstrated high prevalence of conduct disorder, antisocial personality disorder and depression in opioid addicts, and all these neuropsychiatric conditions are characterized by dysfunctional limbic neuronetworks. Although, neuropsychiatric traits are premorbid in many opioid addicts, chronic drug abuse worsens the neuropsychiatric status within the course of the addiction or induces newly developed psychiatric abnormalities.

References

Ballesteros-Yáñez, I., Ambrosio, E., Benavides-Piccione, R., Pérez, J., Torres, I., Miguéns, M., García-Lecumberri, C., DeFelipe, J. The effects of morphine self-administration on cortical pyramidal cell structure in addiction-prone lewis rats. *Cereb. Cortex* 2007;17(1):238-49.

Bauer, L. O. CNS recovery from cocaine, cocaine and alcohol, or opioid dependence: a P300 study. *Clin. Neurophysiol.* 2001;112:1508-15.

Baumgärtner, U., Buchholz, H. G., Bellosevich, A., Magerl, W., Siessmeier, T., Rolke, R., Höhnemann, S., Piel, M., Rösch, F., Wester, H. J., Henriksen, G., Stoeter, P., Bartenstein, P., Treede, R. D., Schrecken-berger, M. High opiate receptor binding potential in the human lateral pain system. *Neuroimage* 2006;30(3):692-9.

Becerra, L., Harter, K., Gonzalez, R. G., Borsook, D. Functional magnetic resonance imaging measures of the effects of morphine on central nervous system circuitry in opioid-naive healthy volunteers. *Anesth. Analg.* 2006; 103(1):208-16.

Beckerman, M. A., Glass, M. J. The NMDA-NR1 receptor subunit and the mu-opioid receptor are expressed in somatodendritic compartments of central nucleus of the amygdala neurons projecting to the bed nucleus of the stria terminalis. *Exp. Neurol.* 2012;234(1):112-26.

Bryun, E. A., Gekht, A. B., Polunina, A. G., Davydov, D. M. Premorbid psychological status in heroin abusers: Impact on treatment compliance. *Zh. Nevrol. Psikhiatr.* Im SS Korsakova 2003;102(6): 21-9.

Castellanos, F. X., Lee, P. P., Sharp, W., Jeffries, N. O., Greenstein, D. K., Clasen, L. S., Blumenthal, J. D., James, R. S., Ebens, C. L., Walter, J. M., Zijdenbos, A., Evans, A. C., Giedd, J. N., Rapoport, J. L. Developmental trajectories of brain volume abnormalities in children and adolescents with attention-deficit/hyperactivity disorder. *JAMA* 2002;288:1740-1748.

Chaves, M. L. F., Bizzi, J. W. J., Palmini, A. L., Izquierdo, I. Naltrexone blocks the enhancing effect of novel experiences on performance in memory tests in humans. *Neuropsychologia* 1988;26(3):491-494.

Chieng, B. C., Christie, M. J., Osborne, P. B. Characterization of neurons *J. Comp. Neurol.* 2006;497(6):910-27.

Cohen, L. J., Gertmenian-King, E., Kunik, L., Weaver, C., London, E. D., Galynker, I. Personality measures in former heroin users receiving methadone or in protracted abstinence from opiates. *Acta Psychiatr. Scand.* 2005;112:149-158.

Daglish, M. R., Weinstein, A., Malizia, A. L., Wilson, S., Melichar, J. K., Britten, S., Brewer, C., Lingford-Hughes, A., Myles, J. S., Grasby, P., Nutt, D. J. Changes in regional cerebral blood flow elicited by craving memories in abstinent opiate-dependent subjects. *Am. J. Psychiatry* 2001; 158(10): 1680-6.

Daglish, M. R., Weinstein, A., Malizia, A. L., Wilson, S., Melichar, J. K., Lingford-Hughes, A., Myles, J. S., Grasby, P., Nutt, D. J. Functional connectivity analysis of the neural circuits of opiate craving: "more" rather than "different"? *Neuroimage* 2003;20(4): 1964-70.

Davids, E., von Bünau, U., Specka, M., Fischer, B., Scherbaum, N., Gastpar, M. History of attention-deficit hyperactivity disorder symptoms and opioid dependence: a controlled study. *Prog. Neuro-Psychopharmacol. Biol. Psychiatry* 2005; 29:291-296.

De Oliveira-Souza, R., Hare, R. D., Bramati, I. E., Garrido, G. J., Azevedo Ignácio, F., Tovar-Moll, F., Moll, J. Psychopathy as a disorder of the moral brain: fronto-temporo-limbic grey matter reductions demonstrated by voxel-based morphometry. *//Neuroimage* 2008. V. 40. № 3. P. 1202-13.

Decety, J., Michalska, K. J., Akitsuki, Y., Lahey, B. B. Atypical empathic responses in adolescents with aggressive conduct disorder: a functional MRI investigation. *Biol. Psychol.* 2009;80:203-11.

Eisch, A. J., Barrot, M., Schad, C. A., Self, D. W., Nestler, E. J. Opiates inhibit neurogenesis in the adult rat hippocampus. *PNAS* 2000; 97(13): 7579-7584.

Evans, J. M., Bey, V., Burkey, A. R., Commons, K. G. Organization of endogenous opioids *J. Comp. Neurol.* 2007;500(3):530-41.

Everitt, B. J., Dickinson, A., Robbins, T. W. The neuropsychological basis of addictive behaviour. *Brain Res. Brain Res. Rev.* 2001;36(2-3):129-38.

Fairchild, G., Passamonti, L., Hurford, G., Hagan, C. C., von dem Hagen, E. A., van Goozen, S. H., Goodyer, I. M., Calder, A. J. Brain structure abnormalities in early-onset and adolescent-onset conduct disorder. *Am. J. Psychiatry* 2011;168: 624-33.

Finger, E. C., Marsh, A. A., Blair, K. S., Reid, M. E., Sims, C., Ng, P., Pine, D. S., Blair, R. J. Disrupted reinforcement signaling in the orbitofrontal cortex and caudate in youths with conduct disorder or oppositional defiant disorder and a high level of psychopathic traits. *Am. J. Psychiatry* 2011; 168:152-62.

Forman, S. D., Dougherty, G. G., Casey, B. J., Siegle, G. J., Braver, T. S., Barch, D. M., Stenger, V. A., Wick-Hull, C., Pisarov, L. A., Lorensen, E. Opiate addicts lack error-dependent activation of rostral anterior cingulate. *Biol. Psychiatry* 2004;55:531-537.

Frick, P. J., Morris, A. S. Temperament and developmental pathways to conduct problems. *J. Clin. Child Adolescent Psychology* 2004;33:54 – 68.

Galynker, I. I., Watras-Ganz, S., Miner, C., Rosenthal, R. N., Des Jarlais, D. C., Richman, B. L., and London, E. Cerebral metabolism in opiate-dependent subjects: effects of methadone maintenance. *Mt. Sinai J. Med.* 2000;67(5-6): 381-7.

Gerra, G., Zaimovic, A., Moi, G., Bussandri, M., Bubici, C., Mossini, M., Raggi, M. A., Brambilla, F. *Prog. Neuro-Psychopharm. Biol. Psychiatry* 2004; 28:129-139.

Gerra, G., Somaini, L., Manfredini, M., Raggi, M. A., Saracino, M. A., Amore, M., Leonardi, C., Cortese, E., Donnini, C. Dysregulated responses to emotions among abstinent heroin users: correlation with childhood neglect and addiction severity. *Prog. Neuro-Psychopharm. Biol. Psychiatry* 2014; 48:220-228.

Harris, G. C., Aston-Jones, G. Altered motivation and learning following opiate withdrawal: evidence for prolonged dysregulation of reward processing. *Neuropsychopharmacology* 2003; 28:865-871.

Hellemans, K. G. C., Everitt, B. J., Lee, J. L. C. Disrupting reconsolidation of conditioned withdrawal memories in the basolateral amygdale reduces suppression of heroin seeking in rats. *J. Neurosc.* 2006; 26:12694-12699.

Hernandez, L. L., Watson, K. L., Fowler, B. M., Bair, K. D., Singha, A. K. Opioid modulation of attention-related responses: peripheral-to-central progression and development of mu influence as learning occurs. *Psychopharmacology* 1997;132:50-60.

Holahan, M. R., Nichol, J., Madularu, D. Spatial information processing consequences of DAMGO injections into the dorsal striatum. *Neurobiol. Learn. Mem.* 2008;90(2):434-42.

Kapoor, R. J., Singh, S. H., Gandhi, A. Autonomic functions and audiovisual reaction time in heroin addicts. *Indian J. Physiol. Pharmacol.* 1993;37; 209-212.

Kennedy, S. E., Koeppe, R. A., Young, E. A., Zubieta, J. K. Dysregulation of endogenous opioid emotion *Arch. Gen. Psychiatry* 2006;63(11):1199-208.

Khalili-Mahani, N., van Osch, M. J., Baerends, E., Soeter, R. P., de Kam, M., Zoethout, R. W., Dahan, A., van Buchem, M. A., van Gerven, J. M., Rombouts, S. A. Pseudocontinuous arterial spin *J. Cereb. Blood Flow Metab.* 2011;31(5):1321-33.

Klega, A., Eberle, T., Buchholz, H. G., Maus, S., Maihöfner, C., Schreckenberger, M., Birklein, F. Central opioidergic neurotransmission in complex regional pain syndrome. *Neurology* 2010;75(2):129-36.

Knoll, A. T., Carlezon, W. A. Jr. Dynorphin, stress *Brain Res.* 2010;1314:56-73.

Koob, G. F., Volkow, N. D. Neurocircuitry of addiction. *Neuropsychopharmacology Reviews* 2010; 35:217-238.

Leppä, M., Korvenoja, A., Carlson, S., Timonen, P., Martinkauppi, S., Ahonen, J., Rosenberg, P. H., Aronen, H. J., Kalso, E. Acute opioid effects on human *Neuroimage* 2006;31(2):661-9.

Le Merrer, J., Becker, J. A., Befort, K., Kieffer, B. L. Reward processing by the opioid system in the brain. *Physiol. Rev.* 2009;89(4):1379-412.

Li, Y. Q., Li, F. Q., Wang, X. Y., Wu, P., Zhao, M., Xu, C. M., Shaham, Y., Lu, L. Central amygdale extracellular signal-regulated kinase signaling pathway is critical to incubation of opiate craving. *J. Neurosci.* 2008; 28: 13248-57.

Ma, N., Liu, Y., Li, N., Wang, C. X., Zhang, H., Jiang, X. F., Xu, H. S., Fu, X. M., Hu, X., Zhang, D. R. Addiction related alteration in resting-state brain connectivity. *Neuroimage* 2010; 49:738-744.

Maarrawi, J., Peyron, R., Mertens, P., Costes, N., Magnin, M., Sindou, M., Laurent, B., Garcia-Larrea, L. Differential brain opioid receptor availability in central and peripheral neuropathic pain. *Pain* 2007; 127(1-2): 183-94.

Mac Intosh, B. J., Pattinson, K. T., Gallichan, D., Ahmad, I., Miller, K. L., Feinberg, D. A., Wise, R. G., Jezzard, P. Measuring the effects of remifentanil on cerebral blood flow and arterial arrival time using 3DG RASE MRI with pulsed arterial spin labeling. *J. Cereb. Blood Flow Metab.* 2008; 28(8):1514-22.

Mahler, S. V., Berridge, K. C. Which cue to "want?" central amygdale opioid activation enhances and focuses incentive salience on a prepotent reward cue. *J. Neurosc.* 2009;29(20):6500-6513.

Mansour, A., Khachaturian, H., Lewis, M. E., Akil, H., Watson, S. J. Anatomy of CNS opioid receptors. *Trends in Neurosciences* 1988;11(7):308 – 314.

Martin-Soelch, C., Chevalley, A. F., Künig, G., Missimer, J., Magyar, S., Mino, A., Schultz, W., Leenders, K. L. Changes in reward-induced brain activation in opiate addicts. *Eur. J. Neurosci.* 2001;14:1360-1368.

Modestin, J., Matutat, B., Würmle, O. Antecedents of opioid dependence and personality disorder: attention-deficit/hyperactivity disorder and conduct disorder. *Eur. Arch. Psychiatry Clin. Neurosci.* 2001; 251:42-47.

Morozov, G. V., Bogolepov, N. N. (1984). *Morphinism*. Moscow: Medicina Publishers.

Mueller, C., Klega, A., Buchholz, H. G., Rolke, R., Magerl, W., Schirrmacher, R., Schirrmacher, E., Birklein, F., Treede, R. D., Schreckenberger, M. Basal opioid receptor binding is associated with differences in sensory perception in healthy human subjects. *NeuroImage* 2010;49:731-737.

Ortiz, J., Raine, A. Heart rate level and antisocial behavior in children and adolescents: a meta-analysis. *J. Am. Acad. Child Adolesc. Psychiatry* 2004;43:154–162.

Passamonti, L., Fairchild, G., Goodyer, I. M., Hurford, G., Hagan, C. C., Rowe, J. B., Calder, A. J. Neural abnormalities in early-onset and adolescence onset conduct disorder. *Arch. Gen. Psychiatry* 2010;67:729-38.

Penney, J. B. Neurochemical Neuroanatomy. In: Fogel, B. S., Schiffer, R. B., Rao, S. M., eds. *Neuropsychiatry.* Williams and Wilkins, 1996: 635-678.

Petrovic, P., Pleger, B., Seymour, B., Klöppel, S., De Martino, B., Critchley, H., Dolan, R. J. Blocking central opiate function modulates hedonic impact and anterior cingulate response to rewards and losses. *J. Neurosci.* 2008;28(42):10509-16.

Prossin, A. R., Love, T. M., Koeppe, R. A., Zubieta, J. K., Silk, K. R. Dysregulation of regional endogenous opioid function in borderline personality disorder. *Am. J. Psychiatry* 2010;167(8):925-33.

Raine, A., Lenez, T., Bihrle, S., LaCasse, L., Colletti, P. Reduced prefrontal gray matter volume and reduced autonomic activity in antisocial personality disorder. *Arch. Gen. Psychiatry* 2000;57:119-127.

Randall-Thompson, J. F., Pescatore, K. A., Unterwald, E. M. A role for delta opioid receptor in the central nucleus of the amygdale in anxiety-like behaviors. *Psychopharmacology* (Berl.) 2010; 212(4):585-95.

Richell, R. A., Mitchell, D. G. V., Newman, C., Leonard, A., Baron-Cohen, S., Blair, R. J. R. Theory of mind and psychopathy: can psychopathic individuals read the 'language of the eyes'? *Neuropsychologia* 2003;41:523–526.

Robinson, T. E., Gorny, G., Savage, V. R., Kolb, B. Widespread but regionally specific effects of experimenter- versus self-administered morphine on dendritic spines in the nucleus accumbens, hippocampus, and neocortex of adult rats. *Synapse* 2002;46:271-279.

Rodefer, J. S., Nguyen, T. N. Naltrexone reverses age-induced cognitive deficits in rats. *Neurobiology of Aging* 2008;29:309-313.

Seidman, L. J., Valera, E. M., Makris, N. Structural brain imaging of Attention-Deficit/Hyperactivity Disorder. *Biol. Psychiatry*; 57:1263-1272.

Schlaepfer, T. E., Strain, E. C., Greenberg, B. D., Preston, K. L., Lancaster, E., Bigelow, G. E., Barta, P. E., Pearlson, G. D. Site of opioid action in the human brain: mu and kappa agonists' subjective and cerebral blood flow effects. *Am. J. Psychiatry* 1998;155(4):470-3.

Schultz, W. The reward signal of midbrain dopamine neurons. *News Physiol. Sci.* 1999; 14: 249-255.

Sim-Selley, L. J., Selley, D. E., Vogt, L. J., Childers, S. R., Martin, T. J. Chronic heroin self-administration desensitizes μ-opioid receptor-activated G-proteins in specific regions of rat brain. *J. Neurosc.* 2000; 20:4555-4562.

Sklair-Tavron, L., Shi, W. X., Lane, S. B., Harris, H. W., Bunney, B. S., Nestler, E. J. Chronic morphine induces visible changes in the morphology of mesolimbic dopamine neurons. *Proc. Natl. Acad. Sci. US 1996;* 93 (20): 11202-7.

Sterzer, P., Stadler, C., Krebs, A., Kleinschmidt, A., Poustka, F. Abnormal neural responses to emotional visual stimuli in adolescents with conduct disorder. *Biol. Psychiatry* 2005;57:7–15.

Sterzer, P., Stadler, C., Poustka, F., Kleinschmidt, A. A structural neural deficit in adolescents with conduct disorder and its association with lack of empathy. *Neuroimage* 2007;37:335-42.

Stevens, M. C., Kaplan, R. F., Bauer, L. O. Relationship of cognitive ability to the developmental course of antisocial behavior in substance-dependent patients. *Prog. Neuro-Psychopharmacol. Biol. Psychiatry* 2001;1523-1536.

Subramaniam, G. A., Stitzer, M. L., Woody, G., Fishman, M. J., Kolodner, K. Clinical characteristics of treatment-seeking adolescents with opioid versus cannabis/alcohol use disorders. *Drug Alcohol Dependence* 2009; 99:141 – 149.

Suh, J. J., Langleben, D. D., Ehrman, R. N., Hakun, J. G., Wang, Z., Li, Y., Busch, S. I., O'Brien, C. P., Childress, A. R. *Drug Alcohol Depend.* 2009; 99:11-17.

Vogt, L. J., Sim-Selley, L. J., Childers, S. R., Wiley, R. G., Vogt, B. A. Colo-colization of μ-opioid receptors and activated g-proteins in rat cingulate cortex. *JPET* 2001;299(3):840-848.

Vogt, B. A., Vogt, L., Farber, N. B. Cingulate cortex and disease models. In: *The rat nervous system*, third edition 2004; 705-727.

Wang, Z. X., Zhang, J. X., Wu, Q. L., Liu, N., Hu, X. P., Chan, R. C. K., Xiao, Z. W. Alterations in the processing of non-drug-related affective stimuli in abstinent heroin addicts. *Neuroimage* 2010; 49:971-976.

Whittington, M. A., Traub, R. D., Faulkner, H. J., Jefferys, J. G. R., Chettiar, K. Morphine disrupts long-range synchrony of gamma oscillations in hippocampal slices. *Proc. Natl. Acad. Sci. US* 1998; 95:5807-5811.

Williams, J. T., Christie, M. J., Manzoni, O. Cellular and synaptic adaptations mediating opioid dependence. *Physiological Reviews* 2001; 81:299-343.

Zijlstra, F., Veltman, D. J., Booij, J., van den Brink, W., Franken, I. H. A. Neurobiological substrates of cue-elicited craving and anhedonia in recently abstinent opioid-dependent males. *Drug Alcohol Depend.* 2009; 99:183-192.

Zubieta, J. K., Ketter, T. A., Bueller, J. A., Xu, Y., Kilbourn, M. R., Young, E. A., Koeppe, R. A. Regulation of human affective responses by anterior cingulate and limbic mu-opioid neurotransmission. *Arch. Gen. Psychiatry* 2003;60(11):1145-53.

Zubieta, J. K., Stohler, C. S. Neurobiological mechanisms of placebo responses. *Ann. NY Acad. Sci.* 2009; 1156:198 – 210.

Index

A

abuse, 58, 67
access, 9, 29, 45
acid, 19, 44, 49, 51
acidic, 43
ACTH, 69
action potential, 12
acute stress, 27
AD, 55, 56
adaptation(s), 43, 52, 55, 76
adductor, 29
adductor longus, 29
ADHD, 65
adhesions, 31
adipose, 26, 27
adipose tissue, 26, 27
adolescents, 38, 71, 72, 74, 76
adrenal gland(s), 54
adrenaline, 42
adrenocorticotropic hormone, 69
adults, 14
affective disorder, 31
age, 20, 65, 75
aggression, 14
agonist, ix, 49, 57, 59, 61, 62, 63, 70
alcohol abuse, 65
alcohol dependence, 24, 34
alcohol use, 76
alkalosis, 23

alters, 44
amino, 49
amplitude, 49
amygdala, vii, viii, 2, 5, 6, 9, 12, 22, 24, 30,
    31, 32, 38, 40, 41, 43, 47, 48, 52, 53, 54,
    55, 56, 57, 58, 60, 61, 63, 69, 71
analgesic, 35
anatomy, 3, 13, 15
anorexia, 45
anterior cingulate cortex, 58, 59, 60, 63, 66,
    68
anterior thalamic nuclei, vii, 3, 6, 40
antisocial behavior, 67, 74, 76
antisocial personality, 58, 65, 66, 67, 70
antisocial personality disorder, 58, 65, 66,
    67, 70
anxiety, 14, 28, 29, 30, 31, 35, 36, 37, 61,
    62, 66, 67, 69, 75
apoptosis, 52
appetite, 42, 45, 48, 49, 56
arousal, 35
arteries, 24
assessment, 15, 17
astrogliosis, 2, 11
ATF, 53
athletes, 33
atrophy, 9, 17, 31
attitudes, 66
autonomic activity, 75
autonomic nervous system, 32

D

E

N